THE
ALLERGY-FRIENDLY
COOKBOOK

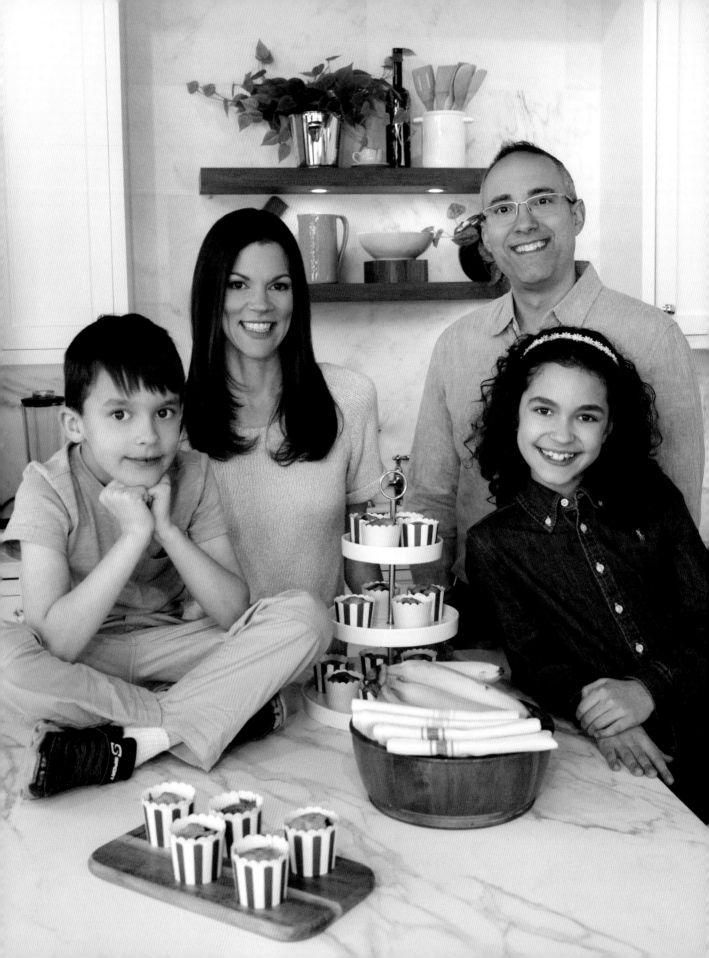

THE ALLERGY-FRIENDLY COOKBOOK

Simple Recipes for the Whole Family

Elizabeth Pecoraro

RED ⚡ LIGHTNING BOOKS

This book is a publication of

RED ⚡ LIGHTNING BOOKS
1320 East 10th Street
Bloomington, Indiana 47405 USA

redlightningbooks.com

© 2023 by Elizabeth Pecoraro

Manufactured in the United States of America

First printing 2023

Cataloging information is available from the Library of Congress.

ISBN 978-1-68435-208-1 (hardback)
ISBN 978-1-68435-210-4 (ebook)

Family photography: Jessie Mignone (@whats_in_westchester_ny).
Styled by Brooke Lawer (@havenbybrooke).
Bilotta Kitchen & Home (@bilottakitchens).

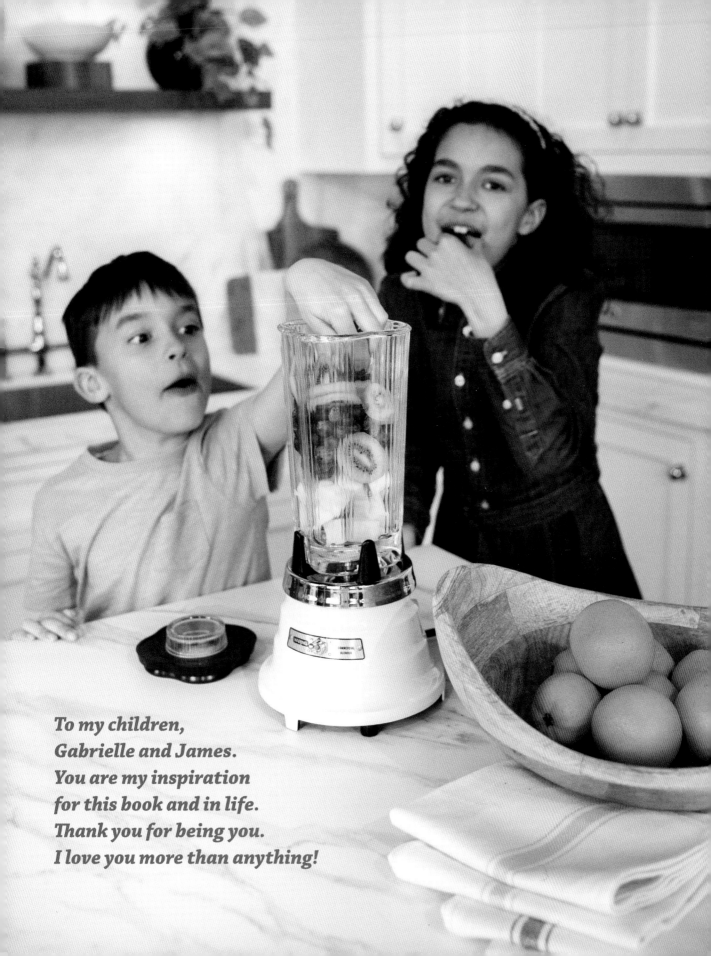

To my children,
Gabrielle and James.
You are my inspiration
for this book and in life.
Thank you for being you.
I love you more than anything!

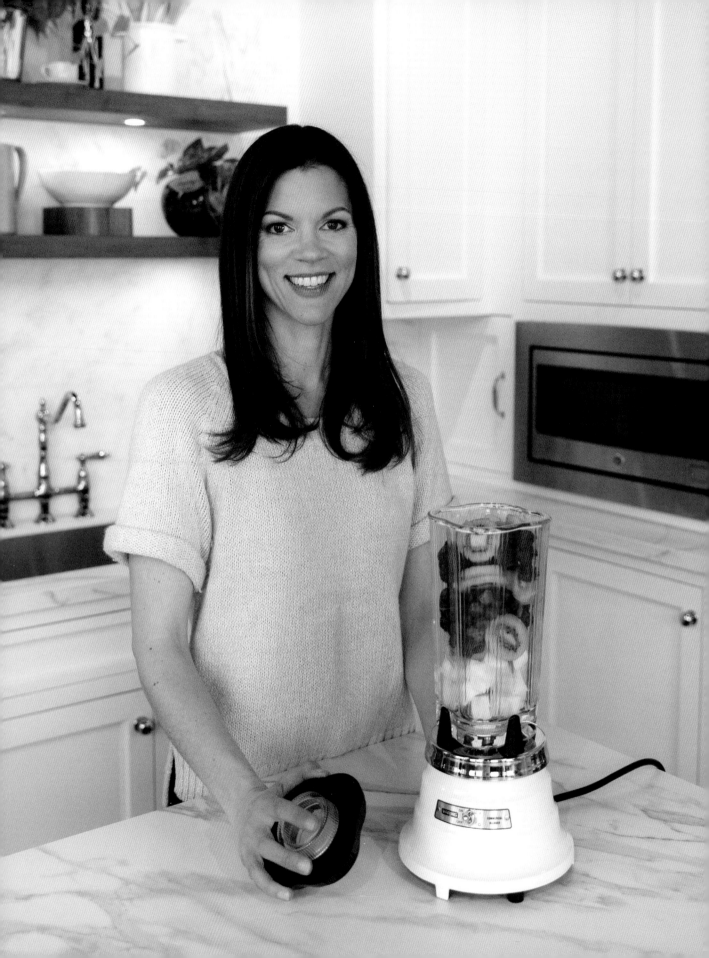

CONTENTS

ACKNOWLEDGMENTS

To everyone at Red Lightning Books who helped perfect this cookbook and get it out to the food allergy community, thank you.

To my fellow food allergy parents, who are up in the middle of the night baking safe treats for their child's school party, who are spending hours at the grocery store checking every label, who are calling manufacturers to find out their allergy protocols, who are packing the entire kitchen when going on vacation, you are inspiring! Thank you.

To the teachers who support the food allergy community and make sure each student stays safe and feels included, thank you.

To my friends, who are always there to give me a high five or a hug, tell me how proud they are of me, let me vent about the latest mom saga, and be my accountability partners, thank you.

To my mom, who is always there for me and has always made me feel that I could accomplish anything, no matter what obstacles were put in front of me, thank you.

To my husband, who has been one of my biggest supporters while I was writing this book. When I was overwhelmed and questioning my ability to complete this project, you would say, "If anyone can do this, you can." Thank you.

Finally, to my children, who deserve the biggest thanks of all. You are the inspiration for this book and the reason I do what I do every day. Always remember that no matter what your dream is, you can achieve it through hard work, determination, and a solid sense of yourself and your mission in life. Put one foot in front of the other, and keep moving forward. You cannot fail if you don't give up. The sky's the limit. Follow your passion!

THE
ALLERGY-FRIENDLY
COOKBOOK

INTRODUCTION

Children with food allergies can sometimes feel left out. Whether with friends, at school or at home, food is at the center of social interaction. For families with food allergies, this can be a challenge, but no one should feel left out when it comes to eating healthy.

As a dietitian who specializes in food allergies, I spend most of my days working one-on-one with parents struggling to make their children safe meals that also meet their nutritional needs. Together, we go through the child's specific food allergies and make a plan to incorporate all the nutrients children need to grow. We also discuss vacations, playdates, meal prep, eating out, trying new foods, and much more. Food allergies impact every aspect of a family's life, and families living with food allergies, first and foremost, need support. This is why I began hosting huddles, which are like support groups, for parents of children with food allergies. We talk about anything food-allergy related, from how to read food labels and shop for groceries to how to talk to family members and friends about food allergies.

Being a food allergy parent myself, I have a certain degree of understanding and empathy that is hard to come by in those not living with food allergies. I have also come across numerous families who have difficulty explaining food allergies to their extended family and friends. It is easy for a parent to get defensive, especially if family members seem to be questioning your child's allergies. I try to take the burden off of the allergy parent and speak with relatives directly. I answer any questions they may have about food allergies and the situation that they see their loved ones in. The truth is, they may not understand the severity of food allergies, and they may even be scared to admit that their grandchild, niece, or nephew could be hurt by food. This is very new for many people, especially for those from older generations. Together, we talk and have an open discussion.

With all my experience as a food allergy mom and dietitian, I asked myself what I would have wanted when my children were first diagnosed. I had many questions, and the allergist couldn't sit with me for hours on end. I had to do a lot of research and talk to several people during this time to get answers, and I was a dietitian! It was all-consuming. What I needed at the time of diagnosis was support and a place where I could get accurate information, recipe ideas, and even access to a medical professional who had time to answer my questions outside of the allergist appointment.

After years of figuring this new life out on my own, I wanted to make it easier for others experiencing the same issues. I also wanted to make sure parents could give their children not only allergy safe options but also healthy ones. So I wrote this cookbook for families living with food allergies—though any family can create and enjoy these healthy recipes as well. These recipes are simple enough for your children to get involved in the kitchen with you, which can inspire their love for cooking. My goal as a mom and nutritionist is to take most of the guesswork out of it for families who are struggling to feed their children with allergies healthy and safe meals. With this cookbook, you can cook healthy meals that are completely free of all top allergens. If I had something like this at the beginning of my food allergy journey, it would have taken some of the initial stress off.

When I set out to write this cookbook, my goal was to create recipes that were allergy-friendly, as well as kid-friendly. I wanted to be sure my children would eat and enjoy every recipe. Therefore, each recipe is kid-approved by my own children. They have even been involved with the creation of these recipes every step of the way.

This book offers sixty allergy-friendly recipes that your whole family will eat and enjoy. The majority are easy enough for you to make in about thirty minutes or less. Of course, desserts and soups always take a little longer due to the baking and cooking time. You shouldn't be spending hours in the kitchen because what parent has time for that? Several of these recipes are based on all-time favorites, but they are revised to make them allergy-friendly and a lot healthier than what you would expect from kid-friendly meals.

As parents to children with food allergies, we are constantly searching for safe foods. Sometimes we go to multiple grocery stores and order online from different manufacturers and allergy-friendly companies. With this cookbook, you will not have to search for special ingredients. The ingredient lists are not pages-long either. The goal is for you to be able to make most of these recipes with foods you already have at home or that you can find easily at any grocery store. You can even grow many of the ingredients in a backyard garden. That is the beauty of a whole-food approach when it comes to cooking, and that is the focus of this book.

Each chapter of the cookbook was chosen for a specific reason. As a dietitian, I get many questions on what parents should feed their children for breakfast, allergies or not. Breakfast can be tricky for a couple of reasons. One is the parents often don't have the time to prepare a healthy breakfast every day, especially when they work. Therefore, I created recipes, such as breads, muffins, and bars, that you can make beforehand. This way, you can just grab and go. I also added some recipes that you can quickly make in the morning.

The second reason breakfast is difficult is that many children don't like traditional breakfast foods, or they only like the options with tons of sugar in them. My breakfast recipes have no added sugar, so parents know their children are getting the nutrition they need without getting loaded up on sugar early in the morning.

Chapter two collects all my family's favorite allergy-friendly soups and starters. Soups are great options when you have limited time during the week. You can batch cook soup on the weekends and freeze leftovers to grab whenever you lack the time to cook from scratch. Also, soups are an easy way to incorporate several nutrients into a meal all at once, compared to putting a plain vegetable on your child's plate that they may not even touch. I also like to pack a thermos filled with soup as a school-lunch option. This makes lunch packing that much quicker, since it is already prepared. Soup also adds variety to the traditional school-lunch sandwich.

When you have food allergies, especially multiple food allergies, it is important to get protein in any way you can. The top nine allergens are mostly protein-rich foods, so when you remove these foods from your child's diet, you are left with few options. Therefore, the nonvegetarian main course recipes in this book tend to use two healthy animal proteins that are not top allergens: turkey and chicken. Also, poultry is versatile and low in saturated fat compared to red meat.

Pasta is my daughter's all-time favorite food, so I included several pasta dishes in this cookbook. If you are living with a gluten allergy, your options for gluten-free pastas are endless. You can opt for pasta made from rice or legumes, such as chickpeas, or even quinoa. Because pasta is also a favorite of many children, learning ways to make traditional favorites, such as lasagna and pasta carbonara, a little healthier and safe was something that was important to me. Many of these pasta recipes, if not all, have a vegetable in them. It may be hidden in some, but you are sure to be giving your child several nutrients in each recipe.

Plant-based diets are also becoming popular these days, for good reason: consuming a plant-based diet, where the majority of your food is from plant sources, is known to be the healthiest way to eat. This doesn't mean you have to become a vegetarian, but focusing on getting your nutrition from nonanimal sources the majority of the time can have benefits. This is why I included a vegetarian section within the main recipes. With a few tweaks, these recipes can easily be vegan as well. When originally creating recipes for my family, they were not always dairy-free because dairy was one of the few allergens we were not allergic to.

Desserts are tough for allergy parents, specifically if there is a nut and/or egg allergy. Eggs are in baked goods. It is that simple. Plus, bakeries tend to have nuts, so the risk of cross contamination is very high. At first, I tried to find premade allergy-friendly baked goods, but due to our numerous allergies and a desire to find options that were not completely laden with sugar, this was not an easy task. I knew I had to start experimenting in the kitchen. There was a lot of trial and error, but now, my children, especially my daughter who has the most allergies, prefers my egg-free baking compared to commercially made baked goods. Also, desserts, of course, have sugar, but allergy-friendly desserts tend to have even more because they try to make up for the altered taste from taking away so many ingredients. If you just add more sugar this makes everything taste better, right? Well maybe, but your child doesn't need tons of sugar with every little treat. My dessert recipes are just the right sweetness to know you are having a dessert without going overboard with sugar.

Throughout the book, you'll notice nutrition notes added to certain recipes that give information on the ingredients in the meals and how they will benefit your health, as well as substitutions, if necessary, in order to make every recipe free of all top nine allergens. You'll also find additional cooking tips, such as ways to switch up the recipe if you are looking for low carb or less sugar or even how to make a sauce into a soup. I hope these tips make this book more personal and helpful to readers.

Last, the appendices at the end of the book include a list of allergy-friendly manufacturers, along with a list of brands our family uses regularly. I have personally checked with every manufacturer, but things change all the time. Call and/or email each company yourself to double-check.

Our Story

The story below is our personal experience. Nothing written here is a recommendation of what you should do with your child. Your specific plan needs to be determined with your pediatrician and allergist.

Gabrielle had her first allergic reaction without us even realizing it. After her first bite of a homemade chocolate cupcake at her first birthday party, she developed a rash on her cheek. I noticed it, but, with food allergies not being top of mind at the time, I shrugged it off. Little did we know that it was an allergic reaction. This was the beginning of a life-changing diagnosis.

At our first allergy appointment with Gabrielle, we found out she tested "positive" for eggs, sesame, peanuts, tree nuts, soy, chickpea, and sunflower seeds, with the peanut allergy being extremely high. We were told to strictly avoid all these foods and come back in one year. A year later, we were in the same office for more tests. The majority of her numbers had gone up— not down, as we'd hoped. The allergist told us that it was not a matter of if she would have an allergic reaction; it was a matter of when. Then the allergist proceeded to tell us that she could not have anything made in a facility with nuts. I would have to contact every manufacturer that didn't label with a "may contain" statement. There would be no eating out at restaurants for now. I would need to inform our family and friends, and when she started school in a couple of months, they would need to understand the severity of her allergies. The allergist prescribed six epi pens (two stay at home, two travel with us, and two are for school).

I remember that moment as clearly as though it were yesterday. I was confused about why this was happening to our child. I never thought this would be her future. I felt defeated and helpless.

School started, and, fortunately for us, the teachers were responsive and took everything I said seriously. Her preschool experience was wonderful. The teachers gave us a heads-up with all food-related parties and projects, and I made substitutions for Gabrielle that were as close to what the other children were having as possible. I have to admit, it was exhausting physically (cooking and baking all the time), mentally, and emotionally. I was constantly worried about the "what ifs." At times, I still am, but those times are farther apart.

When Gabrielle was three years old, I gave birth to her younger brother, James. During the pregnancy, I had no idea what to do. "Should I eat peanuts?" "Should I eat nuts at all?" At the

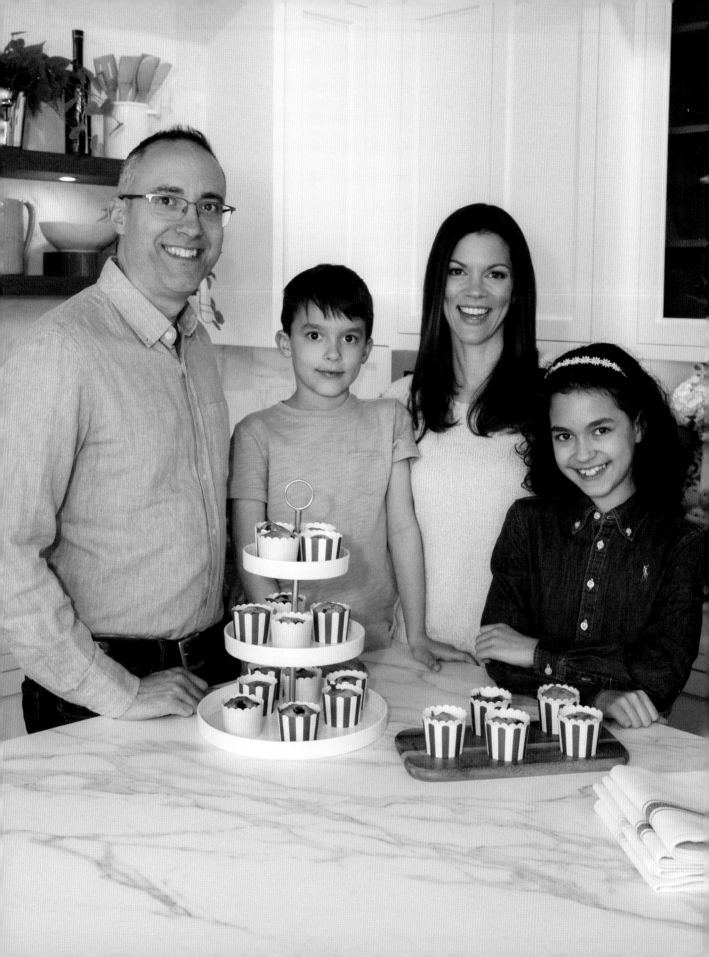

time, the recommendation was not to avoid specific allergens during pregnancy. I couldn't get myself to eat peanuts, but I ate tree nuts and other foods, including Gabrielle's allergens. I delivered a healthy baby boy ten days after Gabrielle's third birthday and began nursing, just as I had with Gabrielle.

Everything was going fine until a couple of months later, when James had blood in his stool. We brought him to the doctor, and he was diagnosed with a milk allergy. I could not believe it. For me, this was worse than being diagnosed with all the other allergies we were already dealing with because this was a different food we had to avoid, and, of course, Gabrielle loved everything dairy. I cried for a long time.

Finally, I got myself together and went to the allergist. This time, I tried someone new. I had begun doing my own research on food allergies, and I wanted a new and fresh perspective, instead of simply being advised to strictly avoid the allergens. Our pediatrician recommended an allergist within their practice. He was very knowledgeable and aggressive with his treatments. He told me that James did have a milk allergy, and I was to avoid dairy in my own diet, since I was nursing. In a couple of months, we could retest for milk, as well as for egg and peanut.

Our appointment finally approached, and they gave James a skin test for peanuts, egg, and milk. He tested borderline positive for all three. His skin test for peanut was smaller than the specific millimeter criteria to be labeled as a definitive allergy. There was a chance he was not allergic. The allergist wanted to challenge James orally to peanut. At first, I thought the man had lost his mind. He saw my face and explained about the new research that involved introducing peanuts to infants in order to decrease their risk of developing an allergy as they grew older. He told us that this could be the only way James would not have to live with a peanut allergy. I agreed, and we scheduled an appointment for a peanut challenge for our seven-month-old baby boy.

The day came for the peanut challenge. James took his first bite and we waited. Nothing happened. The nurse came back with a larger dose. James ate it and seemed to like it, which made things slightly easier. We waited again. No reaction. This went on for two more rounds, and each time the dose was increased. After the last dose, we waited two hours while the nurse and doctor came in and out to check on us. At the end, the allergist came in and said "Congratulations, your son passed his peanut challenge!" I couldn't believe it! I was extremely happy and relieved.

The allergist explained what we needed to do next. He told us that if your infant passes the challenge and a sibling and/or parent has a peanut allergy, the research suggested the child should ingest an infant-safe peanut product three times a week until the age of five. I agreed to doing this. I didn't know how I would do it or how I would keep Gabrielle safe, but I was determined to do whatever it took to help at least one of my children beat a food allergy. After several stressful experiences, we figured out how to give James the peanut product and keep Gabrielle at a safe distance, and then clean everything that could have possibly been exposed.

At this point, we were waiting on the next set of blood results for both of them. We received both good and bad news. James did outgrow his milk allergy and was not allergic to egg either.

Gabrielle's blood test showed that soy had gone up, and she was still high with egg and sesame. In the meantime, the allergist recommended that we challenge her to baked-in egg. At the appointment, they cut the cupcake we brought with us into eight pieces. Gabrielle tasted the cupcake, and said she did not like it. This is a major problem with food challenges. The child has to be willing to eat the food. We begged her to try it and explained, as well as we could to a four-year-old, how this could help her. She agreed to eat it.

Soon after the challenge began, she said her stomach hurt. She went over to the garbage can and threw up. The challenge was over in my eyes. My daughter was having a reaction. The doctor came in again and said he was willing to continue the challenge because there was no rash and she may have thrown up because of nerves. My husband and I decided to stop the challenge. We did not feel comfortable continuing.

We left the allergist and decided to look for someone new once again. As an allergy parent, you need to feel completely comfortable with your allergist and trust them with the safety of your child. I will be forever grateful to him for helping us with James, but his approach didn't feel right to me when it came to Gabrielle.

After some research, we found another allergist. We made an appointment a year later to get both children tested again to see what, if any, changes had happened over the last year.

In the meantime, I gave James hummus because he had eaten chickpea in the past, and, even though Gabrielle was allergic to sesame, it was not a top allergen at the time. Also, the previous doctor hadn't felt testing him for these foods was necessary. The second time he had hummus, there was a reaction just as there had been with Gabrielle.

When the results came back from the new allergist, we found that Gabrielle was not allergic to fish or seafood but had a positive result to coconut, flaxseed, and mustard. Everything else was the same, with soy going up even more. James's results indicated that he was allergic to some tree nuts but not to others, and he had a definite allergy to sesame.

I asked the doctor what our next steps would be with their allergies. She said nothing more at this time. I had been reading research about all the new oral immune therapies, and I was surprised she had not mentioned them. I asked her about everything I had been reading, and she said that if we wanted to go that route, then she recommended going to a food allergy research hospital in the city and that Gabrielle might even be a candidate for research trials. She wrote down the information and I kept that sticky note for almost a year before I made the call.

Seeing the allergist in New York City was a big change. We had to take off work and make a day of it due to the amount of testing and the distance to the hospital. Gabrielle was six, and James was three by this time. We packed up, ready to spend the day in the hospital. They did loads of tests and, at the end of the day, everything was the same with both children, except we added all seeds to Gabrielle's list of allergies. This included flaxseed, hemp, chia, pumpkin, mustard, sunflower, and sesame seed. The good news was that they both had foods that the hospital was willing to challenge. For Gabrielle, we were starting with sunflower, soy, and then baked-in egg again. James would be challenging brazil nut and hazelnut. We were allowed to challenge other tree nuts at home, other than pistachio and cashew, which James was definitely allergic to. Gabrielle was allowed to challenge coconut, poppy seed, and pine nut at home. We went home and waited to be contacted for our in-office challenges.

While we were waiting, I had to find coconut, poppy seeds, and pine nuts that were made in a nut-free facility to eliminate the risk of cross contamination with other tree nuts and peanuts. Coconut and poppy seeds were easy to find, but I had to order pine nuts from a place across the country. In the end, Gabrielle passed all three at-home challenges, and we started to incorporate these food items into her diet.

For James, we had to find walnuts, macadamia nuts, and pecans that were produced in a facility that did not contain any other tree nuts. Phew! The work of an allergy parent is tiring, but we did it. In the end, James passed all his at-home challenges as well.

Finally, they were ready for their first in-office food challenges: sunflower for Gabrielle and brazil nut for James. They both passed! I could not believe it. I finally saw a light at the end of the tunnel. They both had slight positives on their blood tests, but they were not true allergies. I was so happy, I could not put it into words. We incorporated these foods into their diets as well.

Six months later, it was time for the next in-office food challenges. This time it was soy for Gabrielle and hazelnut for James. After the first sip of soy milk, Gabrielle said her throat felt funny. She never complained about her throat during any other reaction in the past. The doctor examined her and said that her throat looked fine and so did her body, and we could keep going. Gabrielle didn't want to take the second dose, but I begged her and tried to explain that this could change her life for the better. She took the dose and again complained about her throat. The doctor said her throat was fine and she was not having a reaction and that we should keep going.

Gabrielle did not want to continue, but I told her she was okay and that she was probably just nervous. We gave her the third dose, and that did it. Gabrielle had a full-on reaction. She knew the whole time. Her body told her immediately that this was not something that was good for her. Part of me wished we listened to her after her first dose, but the other part of me is glad we pushed it because we never would have really known. Soy was out, and we left there deflated but informed.

On a positive note, James passed hazelnut, and we couldn't keep him away from the Nutella.

I never thought Gabrielle would agree to another challenge after that, but when the allergist's office called us for baked-in egg, Gabrielle agreed to go. It had been another six months or so since the soy challenge. She was seven and ready for some more good news. We went with our cupcakes, and it was a difficult task to get her to eat them. She was so used to not eating egg in baked goods that they didn't taste right to her. Even though she did not like it, she finished the challenge and passed. Wow, another success!

The doctor said we needed to wait two hours, and then she would come in with paperwork. Finally, the allergist told us the rules. Gabrielle was to eat baked-in egg every day, if possible. The food item needed to be cooked at 350 degrees for a minimum of thirty minutes, and there couldn't be more than one-quarter of an egg in each serving. "Say what?" I thought I would be able to go to a nut-free bakery and get a cupcake for her. Nope, that was not the case. Once again, I was going to be the at-home baker, and this time, it was not just for a special occasion but all the time.

The doctor said Gabrielle could have a food item from the grocery store where egg was the fourth ingredient or lower on the ingredient label, but, of course, it had to be from a nut-free facility. At this point, my head was spinning, and I couldn't think straight.

The next day, I tried to give Gabrielle that same cupcake recipe that she had at the office. She refused to eat it, so I went to work baking.

This is the point in our story where I realized I could help others with our experience, and I started to write this cookbook. James turned five while I was writing it, and that was the last day we had to give him peanut protein three times per week. I remember when he was seven months old, I was wondering how in the world we would be able to do that until he was five. But we did it, and our son is not allergic to peanuts.

What a ride it has been and still is. Currently, Gabrielle is allergic to peanuts, all tree nuts, soy, egg (not baked-in), and all seeds except sunflower and poppy. She continues to eat baked-in egg, and we have moved on to meatballs with egg and chicken cutlets cooked in an egg wash. We will be heading to the allergist in a couple of months and testing her again to see if egg has come down enough to challenge an actual cooked egg.

We will continue to advocate for the food allergy community and will teach our children how to look out for themselves and others with food allergies, as well as for any person who could be dealing with something you may not see from the outside. It is a long road ahead, but the researchers are amazing, and there are many things in the pipeline. The outlook for children with food allergies is bright.

Now on to the recipes.

Breakfast

Breakfast can be difficult for many parents trying to feed their children wholesome and filling meals. Repetition is a problem, as kids tend to choose one food item that they like and eat this food every morning. Also, breakfast foods that are geared toward children are usually made with tons of added sugar and white starches. They are not good choices to start children's days off right and get them through multiple hours before they eat lunch. Throw food allergies into the mix, and breakfast becomes even harder. Many typical breakfast foods won't work for a family with multiple food allergies. Eggs, muffins, granola, cereal with milk, and yogurt are just a few of the options that could be out if you are a family with multiple food allergies.

In this chapter, I created alternatives to typical breakfast foods that are not only healthy but also kid- and allergy-friendly. Many of them can be made ahead of time and kept in the freezer for easy grab-and-go options.

Personal preferences can make all the difference in whether your child will or will not eat something. Listening to their likes and dislikes will make mealtime a lot easier for you. For example, my son will only eat banana pancakes, but my daughter loves the berry ones, so we split the batter in half and make two different kinds. This is not the biggest deal, and everyone is happy. Small changes to recipes can make a big difference.

The banana avocado breakfast bread was a labor of love. I was determined to make a breakfast bread with zero added sugar. After making the bread probably seven times, we finally figured out the right ratios. This is a great option to freeze to take on vacations or have for breakfast on a busy morning.

Our family loves muffins. They may actually be my favorite food. Traditional muffins are not healthy and contain egg, so I created a couple of egg-free muffin recipes with zero grams of added sugar. The sunflower chocolate chip muffin recipe has one gram of added sugar per muffin but is still, by far, a healthier alternative to other classic chocolate chip muffins. Plus, the sunflower seed butter is a good protein choice that will keep your child satisfied for longer. Muffins are another great option for easy grab-and-go breakfasts. You can make them on the weekend and freeze the leftovers. Take one out of the freezer the night before or pop it in the microwave for fifteen seconds prior to eating. Pair it with a fruit salad and/or spread some vegan butter or other allergy-friendly seed butter on top.

We are also a big smoothie family. We either have smoothies at breakfast or as an afternoon snack. Adding seed butter or dairy-free yogurt will increase the protein and make this smoothie thicker and more substantial. My children prefer to have the smoothie without added protein and drink it with a protein-rich food, such as toast and seed butter or a protein waffle, instead. Smoothies after school fill children up enough so they won't continue snacking on unhealthy choices right before dinner.

Finally, oatmeal sometimes gets a bad rap as being boring, but not with the "elevated" version in this book. Children love to choose their own toppings to create their own personal oatmeal. Put out a number of topping options, and let them go to town. They will get in additional nutrients and fiber with the fresh- and dried-fruit toppings.

Avocado Toast

Prep Time: 5 minutes

INGREDIENTS

1 slice bread*

¼ avocado

¼ tsp olive oil

¼ tsp balsamic vinegar (optional)

Salt and pepper, to taste

DIRECTIONS

1. Toast bread.*

2. Spread avocado on toast.

3. Drizzle with olive oil and vinegar, if using.

4. Sprinkle with salt and pepper.

COOKING TIP
You can also add sliced tomato, strawberries, or a protein such as turkey bacon or ham. If not allergic, an over-easy egg or sliced hard-boiled egg also makes a great addition.

NUTRITION NOTE
Avocado toast was very popular for a while, but the fad seems to be fading. Don't let it! Avocados are a great source of potassium, and they are packed with monounsaturated fats, high in fiber, and rich in folate. This is one fruit you do not want to skip.

*See the appendix for allergy-friendly alternatives.

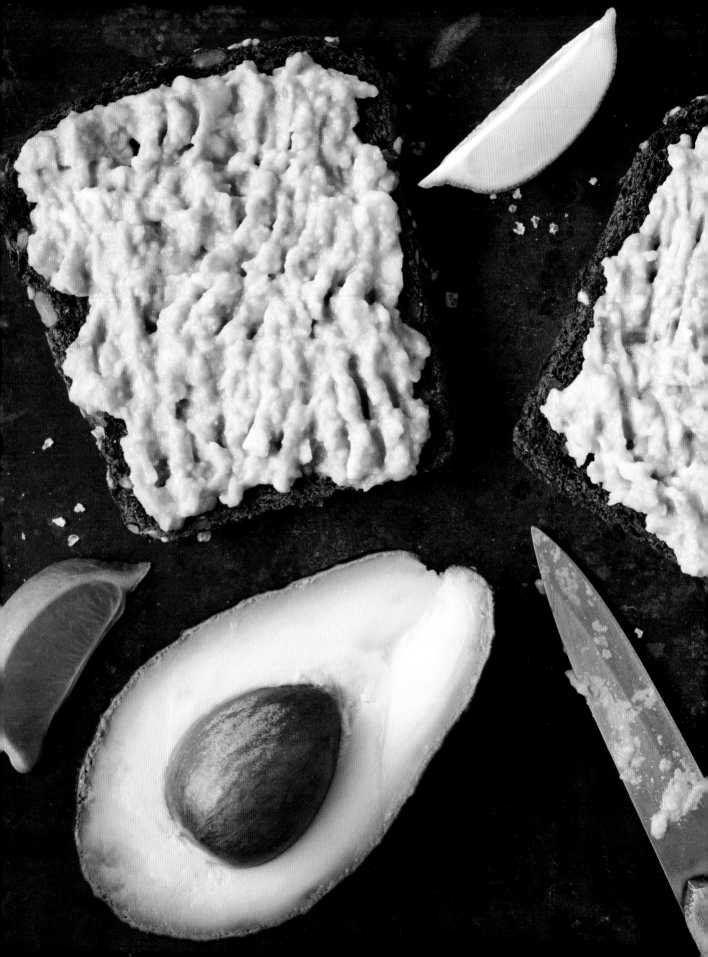

Banana Avocado Breakfast Bread

Prep Time: 15 minutes
Cook Time: 1 hour

INGREDIENTS

2 cups flour*

2 tsp baking powder

1 tsp baking soda

2 tsp cinnamon

¼ tsp salt

3 very ripe medium-sized bananas
   (this is your only source of sweetness,
   so the riper, the better)

½ medium ripe avocado

¼ cup milk or milk substitute*

1 tsp lemon juice

1 tsp vanilla extract

¼ cup avocado oil

1 tsp oil (to coat loaf pan)

DIRECTIONS

1. Preheat oven to 350 degrees.

2. Combine dry ingredients (flour,* baking powder, baking soda, cinnamon, and salt) into a medium-sized bowl. Whisk until combined.

3. Mash bananas in a large bowl. Add avocado and combine thoroughly.

4. Add milk,* lemon juice, vanilla, and oil to the bowl. Blend. Use a mixer to get it smooth.

5. Add dry ingredients to wet ingredients one-third at a time. Stir until just combined each time. You do not want to overmix, or the bread will get chewy.

6. Coat loaf pan with cooking spray or oil. Pour batter into loaf pan.

7. Bake at 350 degrees for 50 minutes to 1 hour or until a toothpick inserted in the center comes out clean.

8. Let cool for at least 10 minutes and remove from pan.

COOKING TIP

You will know the avocado is ripe when it begins to blacken and is somewhat soft—not mushy—to the touch. Wash your avocado before cutting into it.

NUTRITION NOTE

There is no added sugar in this recipe, so it can be a great breakfast option for you and your children, especially with the added healthy fat from the avocado. If you want more sweetness, add sugar, but by doing this, you will be creating more of a dessert than a breakfast. If adding sugar, start with ¼ cup, and see how little you really need. Most banana bread recipes have at least 1 cup of sugar in them. You do not need this much. Also, mini chocolate chips would be a delicious addition.

*See the appendix for allergy-friendly alternatives.

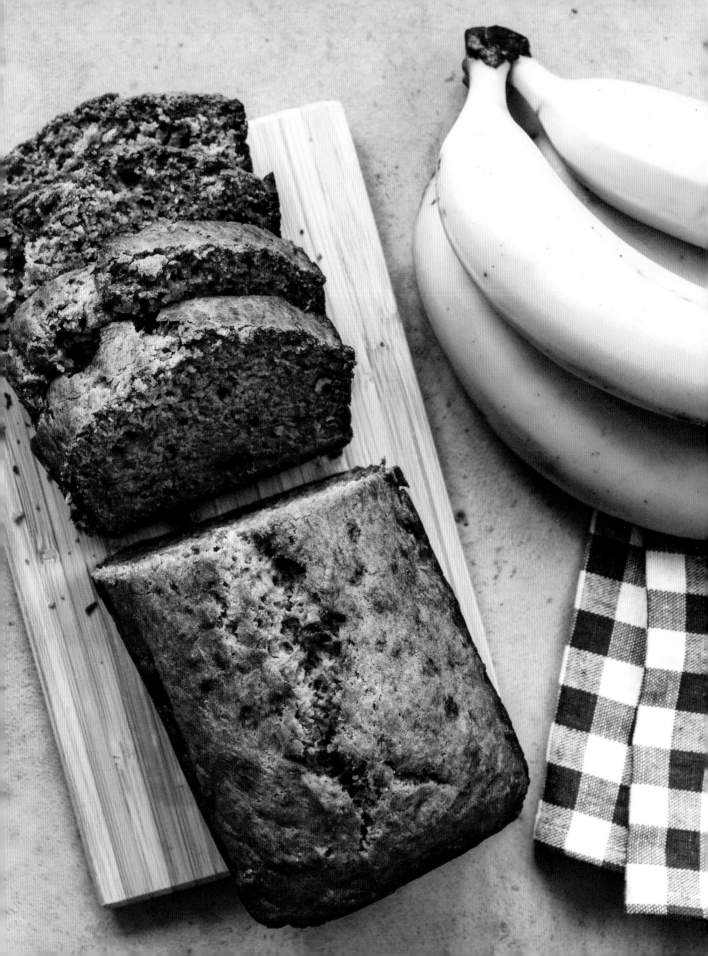

Banana Muffins

Makes 12 muffins.
Prep Time: 10 minutes
Cook Time: 20 minutes

INGREDIENTS

1½ cups whole oat flour

1 tsp baking powder

1 tsp baking soda

1 tsp cinnamon

⅛ tsp salt

3 very ripe bananas

⅓ cup oil

1 tsp vanilla extract

DIRECTIONS

1. Preheat oven to 375 degrees.

2. Line a muffin tin with liners.

3. Combine dry ingredients (oat flour, baking powder, baking soda, cinnamon, and salt) in a small bowl.

4. In a mixing bowl, mash the bananas with a large fork. Add oil and vanilla extract and combine well.

5. Add dry ingredients to wet ingredients and mix until just combined.

6. Scoop batter into cupcake liners.

7. Bake for 20 minutes or until top is golden brown.

COOKING TIP

To make oat flour, put 1½ cups oats in a food processor and blend. Feel free to add fresh blueberries to this recipe as well. Delicious!

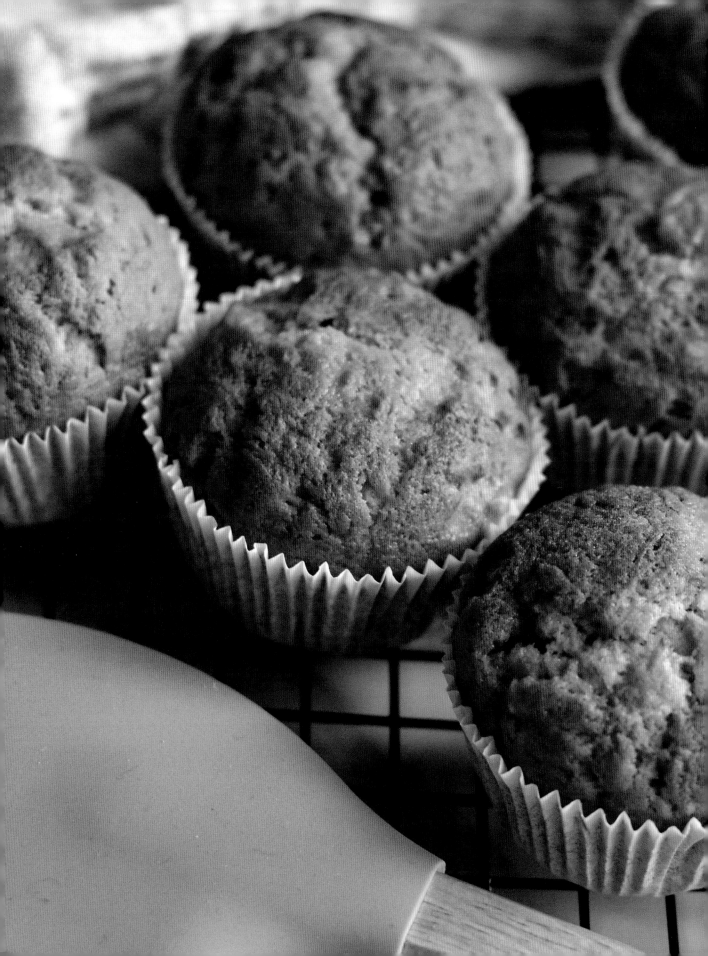

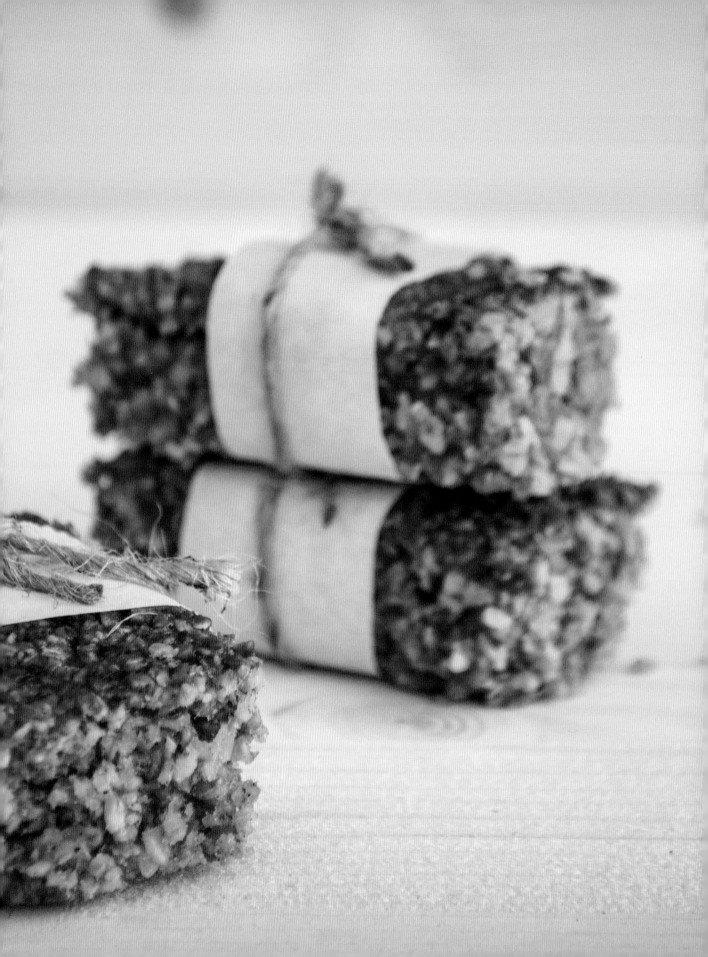

Banana Oatmeal Breakfast Bars

Makes 9 bars.
Prep Time: 10 minutes
Cook Time: 30–40 minutes

INGREDIENTS

2 cups oats

1½ tsp baking powder

⅛ tsp salt

1 tsp cinnamon

2 very ripe bananas

1 cup milk or milk substitute*

½ cup unsweetened applesauce

1 tsp vanilla extract

DIRECTIONS

1. Preheat oven to 350 degrees.

2. In a medium-sized bowl, combine dry ingredients (oats, baking powder, salt, and cinnamon).

3. In a large bowl, mash up bananas with a fork and add wet ingredients (milk,* applesauce, and vanilla). Mix until combined.

4. Add dry ingredients to wet and combine.

5. Spread oat mixture into a greased 8 × 10 or 9 × 9 baking dish.

6. Bake for 30–40 minutes.

COOKING TIP

If you want to make this a little sweeter or have more of a granola-breakfast-bar feel, add mini chocolate chips and/or raisins. Just remember that the more chips you add, the higher your sugar intake.

*See the appendix for allergy-friendly alternatives.

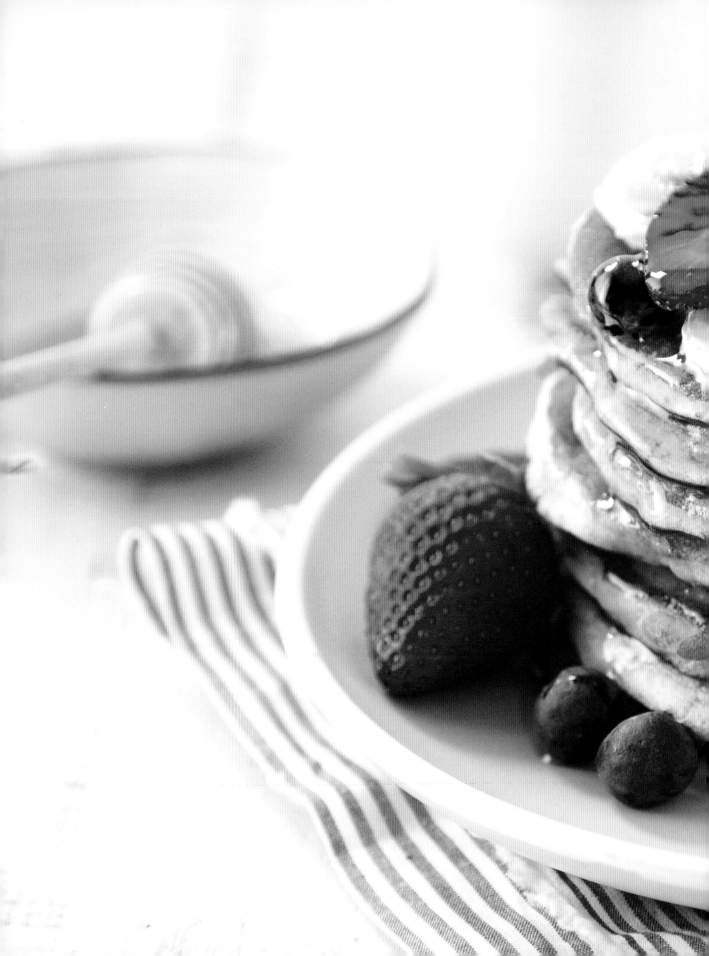

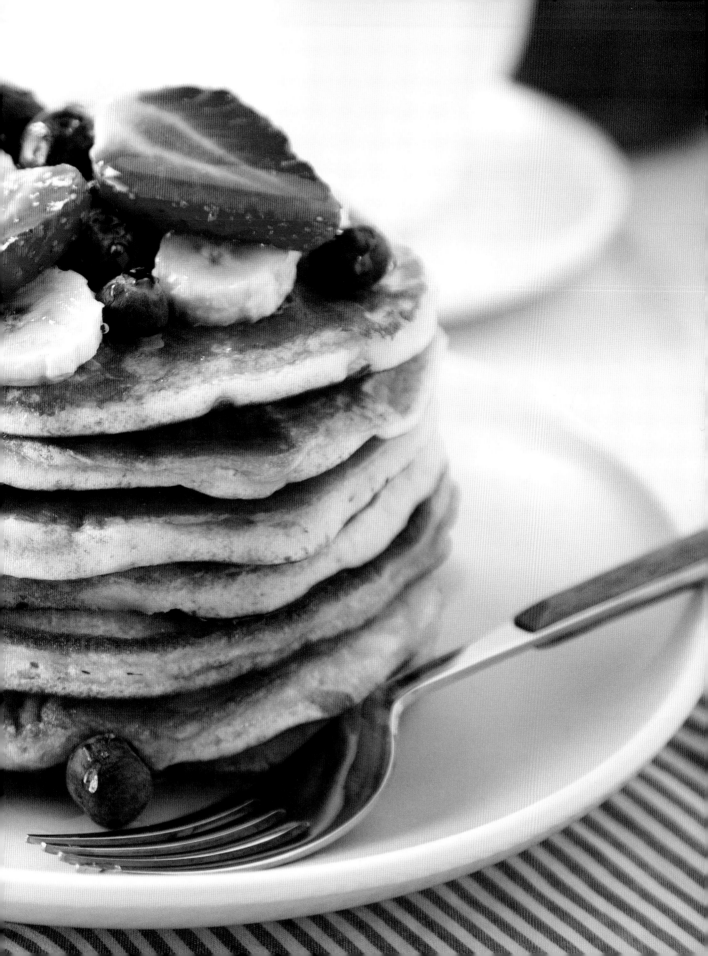

Berry Pancakes

Makes 10–12 pancakes.
Prep Time: 5 minutes
Cook Time: 15 minutes

INGREDIENTS

2 cups flour*

1 T baking powder

½ tsp salt

1½ cups milk or milk substitute*

½ cup unsweetened applesauce

2 tsp cinnamon

1½ cups frozen or fresh blueberries and strawberries (defrost frozen berries first)

DIRECTIONS

1. Mix all ingredients in a bowl.

2. Heat a nonstick pan to low/medium heat.

3. Scoop a large spoonful of batter into pan. When bubbles begin to form, flip over the pancake.

4. Repeat step three until all batter is used.

COOKING TIP

To switch it up, try a different assortment of fruits in these pancakes. To make them sweeter, add banana.

*See the appendix for allergy-friendly alternatives.

Fruit Smoothie

Makes a single 12-oz serving.
Prep Time: 5 minutes.

INGREDIENTS

1 ripe banana

½ cup frozen strawberries

½ cup frozen blueberries

1 large handful of baby spinach

6 oz cold water

DIRECTIONS

Add all ingredients to the blender and blend until smooth. Add more water for desired consistency.

NUTRITION NOTE

This smoothie is a great way to get fruits and veggies into your child's diet without fuss. This smoothie tastes great, contains only natural sugar, and packs in a ton of vitamins and fiber. For added protein, add ground seeds—if your child does not have an allergy—such as hemp, flax, or chia.

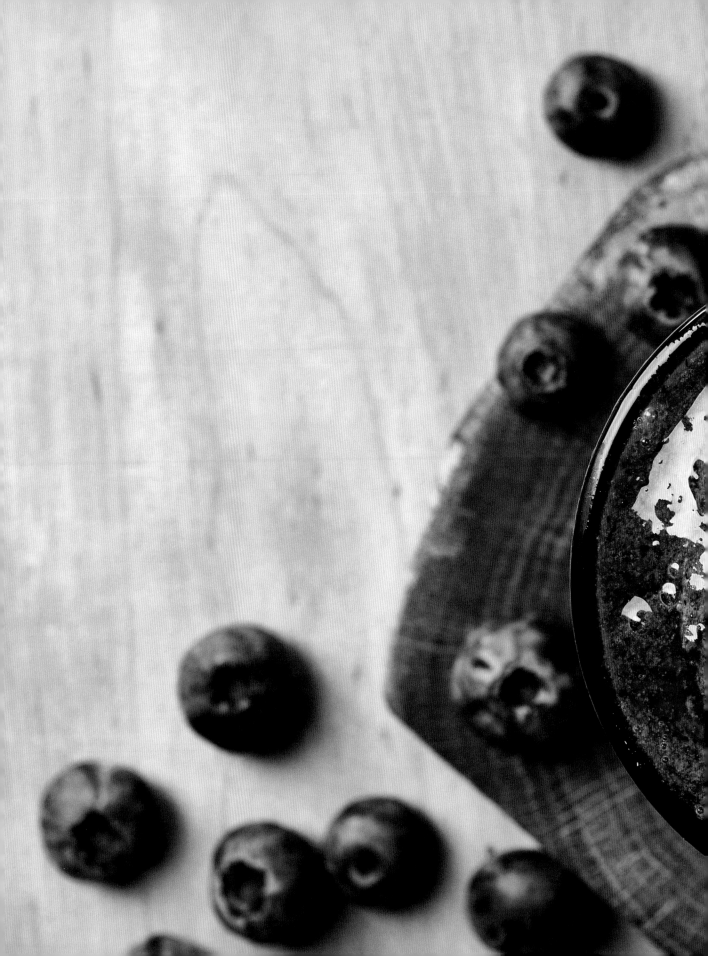

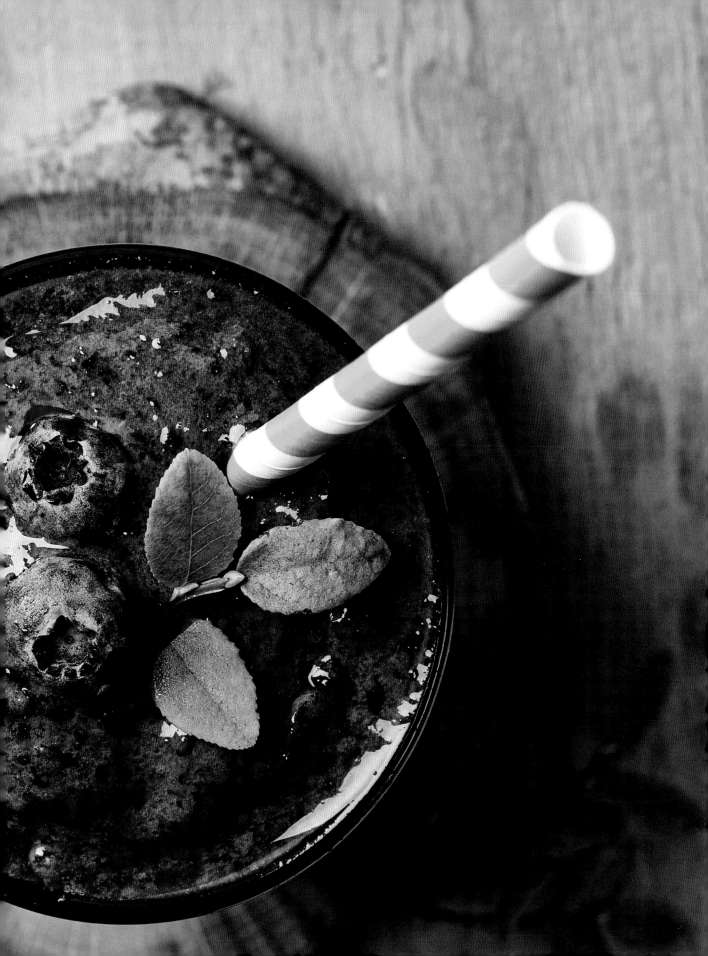

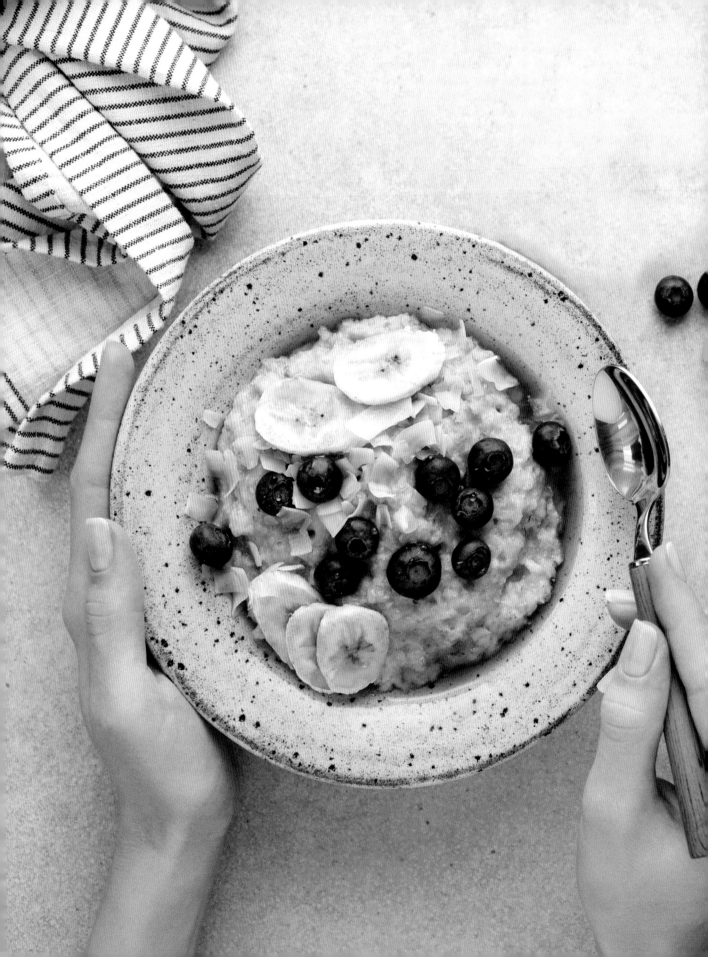

"Elevated" Oatmeal

Makes 1 serving.
Prep Time: 5 minutes
Cook Time: 1 minute

INGREDIENTS

½ cup dry oats

⅔ cup water, milk, or milk substitute*

½ banana, sliced

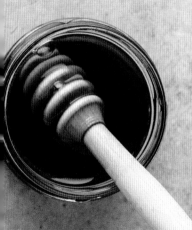

DIRECTIONS

1. Put all ingredients in a microwave-safe bowl and cook on high for 1 minute.

2. Mix.

3. Add additional toppings, as desired. These can include:

   ¼ cup blueberries

   ¼ cup strawberries

   ¼ cup mango chunks

   2 dates, chopped

   15–20 raisins

   1 tsp cinnamon

   coconut flakes

COOKING TIP

If oatmeal is too thick, add a drop of liquid. If too thin, put back in the microwave for an additional 15 seconds.

NUTRITION NOTE

A plain bowl of oatmeal can get very boring, but once you incorporate fun toppings, it changes completely. Plus, you are adding tons of nutrients to your breakfast as well.

*See the appendix for allergy-friendly alternatives.

Sunflower Chocolate Chip Oatmeal Muffins

Makes approximately 20 muffins.
Prep Time: 10 minutes
Cook Time: 25 minutes

INGREDIENTS

3 ripe bananas

1 cup milk or milk substitute*

½ cup no-sugar-added sunflower butter

½ cup unsweetened applesauce

3 cups oats

3 T chocolate chips*

1 T baking powder

1 tsp vanilla

DIRECTIONS

1. Preheat oven to 350 degrees.

2. Line muffin tin with foil liners.

3. In a medium-sized mixing bowl, mash bananas with a fork. Add the rest of the ingredients and stir.

4. Fill each liner almost to the top with batter.

5. Bake for 25 minutes or until baked through. Do the toothpick test.

COOKING TIP

Toothpick test: Stick a toothpick into one of the center muffins and see if it comes out clean. If there is batter on the toothpick, continue baking for 2–3 minutes more, and check again. This batter has a lot of moisture, so foil liners are important.

Also, since this recipe makes a bunch, freeze leftovers, and then pop them in the oven or microwave to warm up before eating.

NUTRITION NOTE

These are dense muffins due to the oats and sunflower butter as well as the lack of eggs. They are not as light as regular muffins and could easily be turned into bars. The added sugar is minor and accounts for only 1 gram of added sugar per muffin, unless you add more chocolate chips.

*See the appendix for allergy-friendly alternatives.

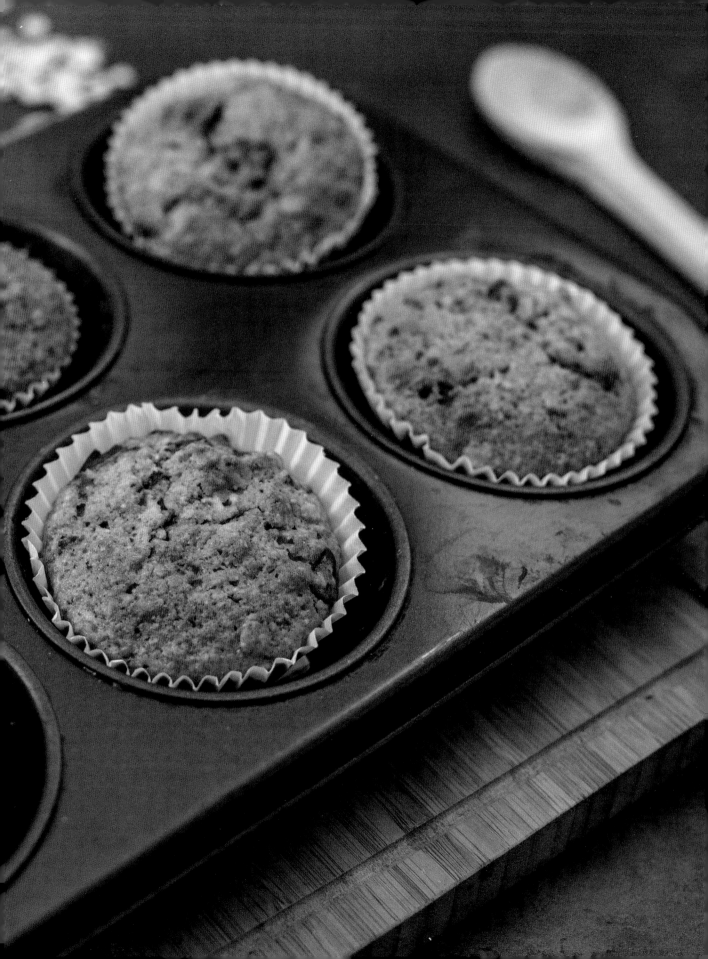

Soups and Starters

Soups are a great way to get several nutrients into your diet and are a wonderful alternative to the traditional salad or side of broccoli. They may take a little additional time to prepare but are worth it in the end. Once the ingredients are in the pot, the rest is done for you. Make a big pot of soup on Sunday and portion it out for the week or freeze the leftovers and have it whenever you feel like it. These soup recipes are not only packed with flavor but also tons of vitamins and minerals. I love making the crockpot chicken chili on cold winter days when I don't have a lot of time. I just throw everything into the slow cooker for six hours, and voilà! Dinner is served. Nan's turkey vegetable soup is another favorite of mine because my grandmother created the original recipe. I made a few tweaks to her recipe to fit our family's needs and came out with a delicious, safe and healthy ground turkey soup recipe.

During the summer, we always grow tons of zucchini. If I am not making the zucchini bread in this cookbook, then I'm making the zucchini soup. It is very light, so it is a great start to any meal. Chicken noodle soup is my children's favorite. They always ask for it when they aren't feeling well and sometimes randomly ask me to cook up a batch just because. It is such a great way to get in veggies, protein, and a whole-grain starch while hydrating them.

The lentil soup recipe is really simple and absolutely delicious! It is packed with fiber and is a meal by itself. I make this recipe all the time as a lunch option for my children and me. I freeze the leftovers for a quick and easy lunch to pack on busy work days. As a child, I always loved tomato soup and grilled cheese. I wanted to create a tomato soup with less sodium than the canned varieties, as well as a dairy-free option. It took me a little while to perfect, but this is a hit with the kids and my husband. When the family sees me making tomato soup, they know that grilled cheese is coming their way too. For those living with a dairy allergy, the appendix lists great alternatives for cheese.

When we have guests, we love to put out starters. The recipes in this chapter are our favorite appetizers when we have gatherings with friends and family. As a child and young adult, I never liked guacamole. The store-bought kinds didn't taste good to me. Then food allergies came into my family's life, and I wanted my daughter to have avocado in different ways. I experimented with my own guacamole recipe, and I have been told time and time again that this is the best guacamole our friends have ever had. As far as hummus goes, this is a food that my husband and I loved to eat prior to having children. Also, I gave each of my children hummus before knowing they had a sesame allergy. They both had it the first time with no problem, and they loved it. Both of them had reactions the second time I offered them hummus. I decided to make a tahini-free version, so we can all enjoy hummus with veggies as a family. The zucchini bites are a big hit with adults and children. They are full of flavor and, of course, nutrients from the zucchini. This is a starter we can't refill quickly enough.

Chicken Noodle Soup

Prep Time: 15 minutes
Cook Time: 4 hours (if using slow cooker to cook chicken)

INGREDIENTS

2 boneless, skinless chicken breasts

1 cup of water or chicken broth for cooking chicken in slow cooker

1 T oil

2 garlic cloves, minced

½ yellow onion, diced

4 stalks celery cut into ½-inch pieces

4 carrots, cut into thin disks

1 box (32 oz) of low-sodium chicken broth

4 cups water

½ lb pasta*

DIRECTIONS

1. Place the chicken breasts into a slow cooker on high for four hours with 1 cup of water or chicken broth.

2. When chicken has 30 minutes left to cook, heat oil in a large soup pot and sauté garlic, onion, celery, and carrots for about 5 minutes, stirring often.

3. Add 32 oz (1 box) of low-sodium chicken broth and 4 cups water to pot. Simmer for 10 minutes.

4. Add pasta* to pot and cook until tender (about 8 minutes).

5. When chicken is cooked, shred and add to the pot.

COOKING TIP

This is a great recipe to make using leftover chicken. This way, the first step is done for you. You can also use a rotisserie chicken if you don't have time for the slow cooker. The benefit of the slow cooker is how tender the chicken gets, and depending on the preparation method, a rotisserie chicken may not be safe for certain food allergies.

NUTRITION NOTE

Why chicken soup for a cold? Studies suggest the hot fluids help increase the movement of nasal mucus and improve the function of protective cilia, the tiny hair-like projections in the nose that prevent contagions from entering the body. None of the research is conclusive; however, at the very least, chicken soup with vegetables contains lots of healthy nutrients, increases hydration and tastes good, too.

*See the appendix for allergy-friendly alternatives.

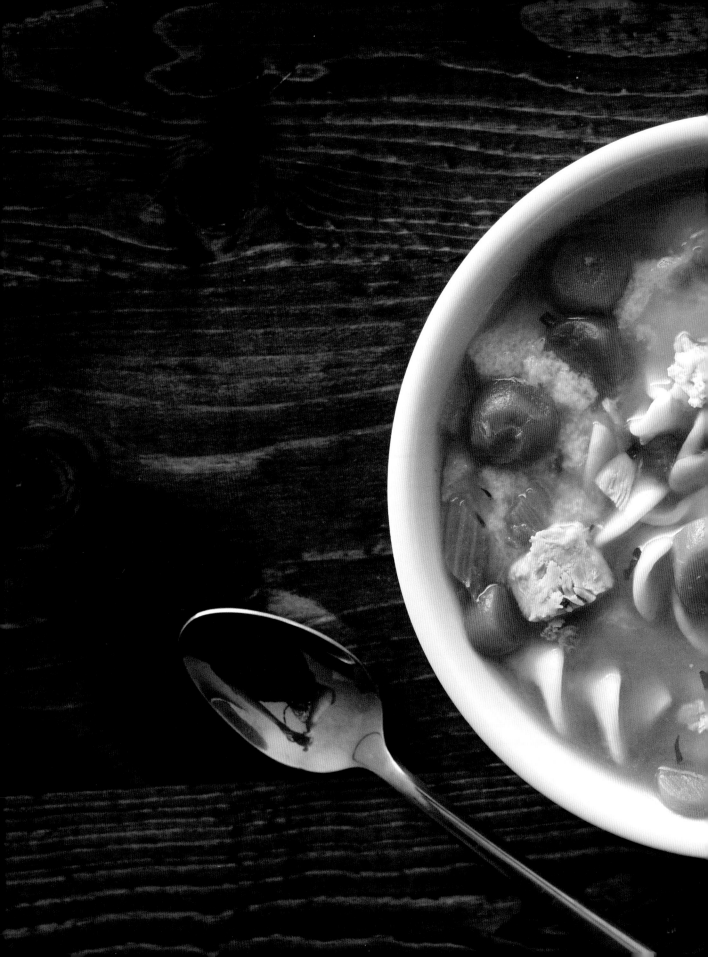

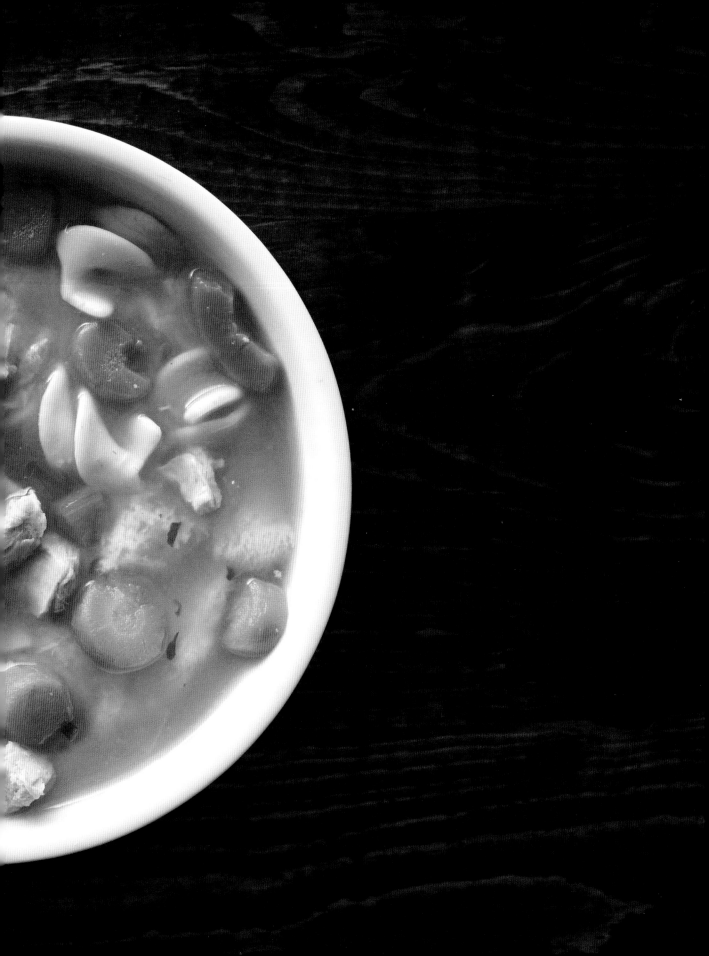

Crockpot Chicken Chili

Prep Time: 15 minutes
Cook Time: 4–6 hours

INGREDIENTS

2–3 boneless, skinless, chicken breasts

1 small yellow onion, chopped

1 red bell pepper, chopped

1 15-oz can of cannellini beans, rinsed and drained

1 15-oz can of kidney beans, rinsed and drained

1 15-oz can of diced tomatoes

2 cups chunky tomato sauce

1 tsp chili powder

1 tsp ground cumin

1 tsp ground ginger

1 tsp turmeric

Salt and pepper, to taste

2 bay leaves

Shredded cheddar cheese*

3–4 slices of avocado

DIRECTIONS

1. Place all ingredients (except cheese* and avocado) into a slow cooker.

2. Stir ingredients together.

3. Cover and cook on high for 4 hours or low for 6 hours.

4. Remove bay leaves.

5. Pull chicken apart with two forks until shredded. Stir all ingredients until combined.

6. Sprinkle shredded cheese* and sliced avocado on top when serving.

NUTRITION NOTE

Cumin is very dense in iron, providing almost 20 percent of your daily iron in one teaspoon.

*See the appendix for allergy-friendly alternatives.

Nan's Turkey Vegetable Soup

Prep Time: 20 minutes
Cook Time: 1 hour and 10 minutes

INGREDIENTS

2 large carrots, sliced into disks

1 red pepper, chopped into bite-sized pieces

4 celery stalks, chopped into bite-sized pieces

1 25-oz jar of tomato basil tomato sauce

2 cups water

1 T oil

1 yellow onion, chopped

1 lb lean (93/7) ground turkey

1 15-oz can of kidney beans

1 T oregano

1 T onion powder

1 T garlic powder

DIRECTIONS

1. Place carrots, peppers, celery, sauce, and water in a large pot. Bring to a boil.

2. While veggies are cooking, sauté onion in oil for 2 minutes.

3. Add ground turkey to onion. Chop up turkey and cook until browned (5–7 minutes.)

4. Turn veggies down to a simmer; add kidney beans, oregano, onion powder, and garlic powder.

5. Add ground turkey and onion mixture to pot.

6. Cover and simmer for 1 hour. Serve.

NUTRITION NOTE

We never add any salt to this soup because the seasonings give it so much flavor. If you must add salt, start with a small amount to see if that will do the trick.

Nan's Soup is a recipe my grandmother created. It is closer to a chili than a soup, but this is what we have always called it, and so I wanted to stick with the name. Originally, this recipe called for the addition of rice, but I didn't have any the first time I made it, so I skipped it, and my family ended up loving it just as much. If you want to make this recipe even heartier, add some rice, just like Nan would do.

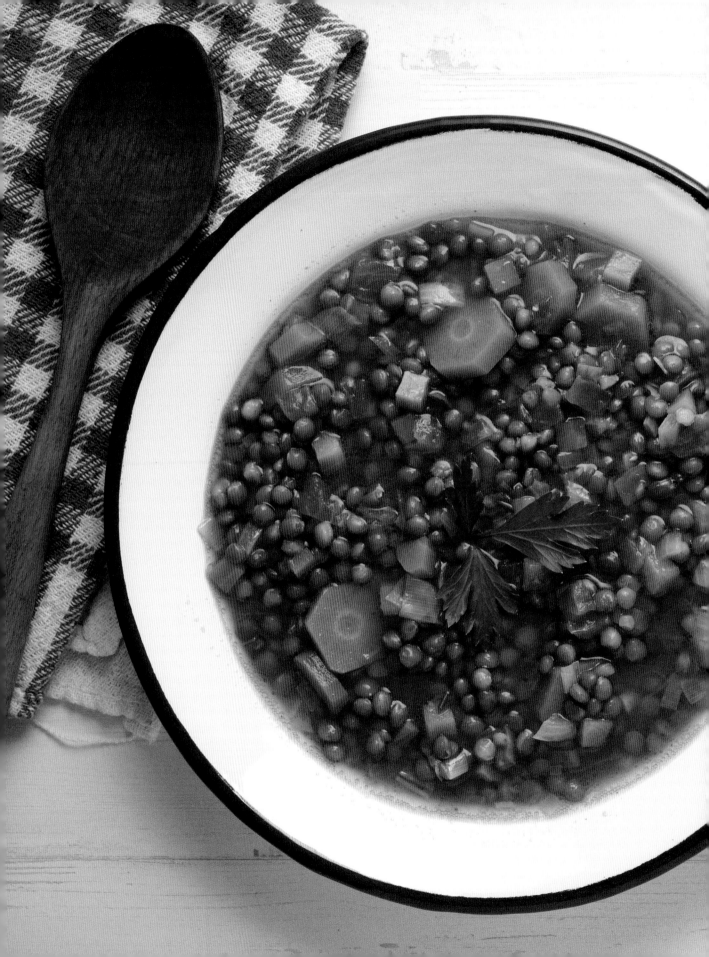

Lentil Soup

Prep Time: 15 minutes
Cook Time: 35 minutes

INGREDIENTS

1 T of oil

4 garlic cloves, minced

1 small white onion, finely chopped

1 large carrot, cut into thin disks

3 celery stalks, chopped

2 cups dried red lentils
(rinse lentils prior to cooking)

1 15-oz can of fire-roasted
diced tomatoes

6 cups low-sodium chicken or
vegetable broth

1 tsp cumin

2 dried bay leaves

DIRECTIONS

1. Heat oil in a large pot over low heat. Add garlic and onion, and cook for 2 minutes.

2. Add carrot and celery. Cook until softened (about 5 minutes).

3. Add all remaining ingredients. Stir.

4. Increase heat, and bring to a boil. Cover and turn down heat to a simmer. Simmer for 25–30 minutes or until lentils are soft.

5. Remove bay leaves, and season with salt and pepper.

NUTRITION NOTE

Lentils are a great source of folate and fiber. The most commonly used lentils for soups are red lentils, since they have a soft texture when cooked. Brown lentils have a mild, earthy flavor; green, a slightly peppery flavor; and yellow lentils have a sweet, nutty flavor.

Tomato Soup

Prep Time: 10 minutes
Cook Time: 15 minutes

INGREDIENTS

1 T oil

1 small white onion, chopped

2 garlic cloves, minced

2 15-oz cans of fire-roasted crushed tomatoes

1 cup shredded cheddar cheese*

½ cup chopped fresh basil

1 T sugar

DIRECTIONS

1. Heat oil in a large pot over low/medium heat.

2. Sauté onion and garlic until onion is somewhat soft (about 4 minutes).

3. Add tomatoes, cheese,* basil, and sugar to pot. Bring to a boil.

4. Put everything into a blender or food processor, and blend until smooth.

COOKING TIP

Adding a little sugar cuts the acidity of the tomatoes. Feel free to add a milk substitute of choice for an even creamier version.

NUTRITION NOTE

Since heat processing increases the antioxidant and lycopene levels of tomatoes, cooking them boosts their cancer-fighting ability.

*See the appendix for allergy-friendly alternatives.

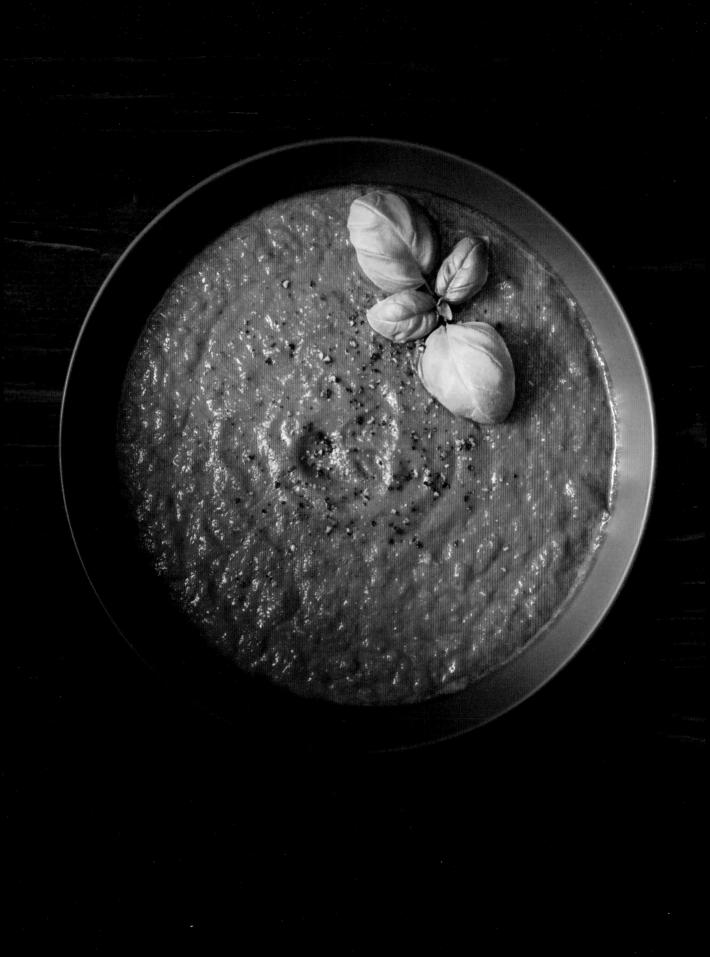

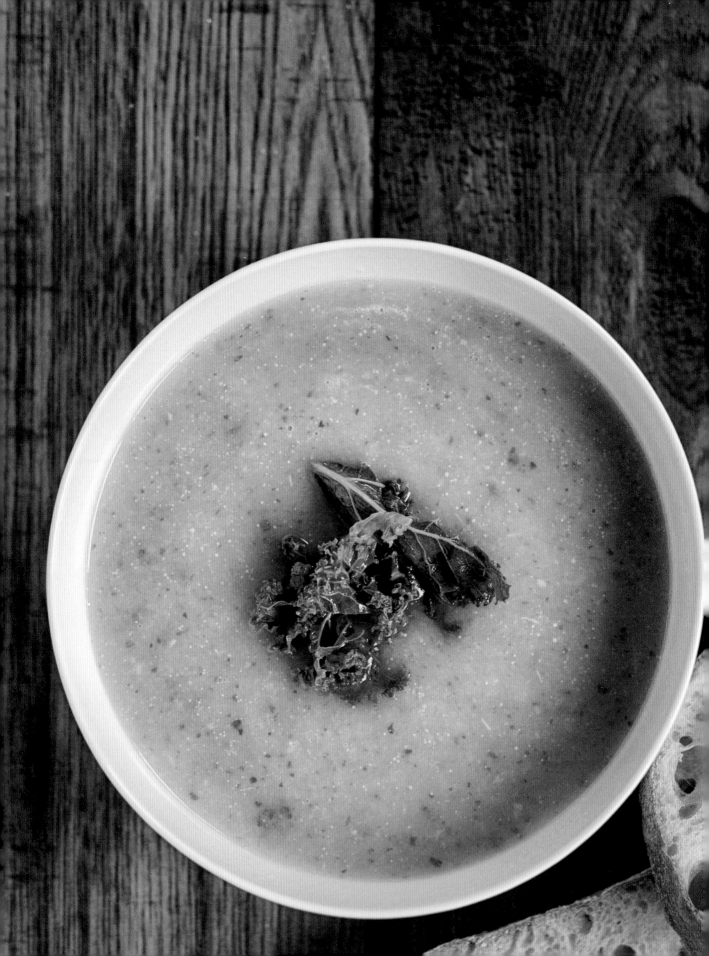

Zucchini Soup

Prep Time: 15 minutes
Cook Time: 20 minutes

INGREDIENTS

4 zucchinis, grated

1 T olive oil

1 T dairy-free butter*

1 medium yellow onion, chopped

1 garlic clove, minced

1–2 cups low-sodium vegetable broth

Salt and pepper, to taste

DIRECTIONS

1. Grate zucchini.

2. Lay out grated zucchini, and use paper towels to remove any excess moisture. You may have to do this a couple of times to get out as much water as possible.

3. Heat oil and butter* over low/medium heat in a large sauté pan, and sauté onion and garlic for about 2 minutes, stirring occasionally.

4. Add grated zucchini and stir. Cover pan, and lower heat. Cook for about 10 minutes.

5. Put zucchini mixture into a food processor, and blend until smooth.

6. Add ½ cup of vegetable broth and blend. Keep doing this with ½ cup broth until you reach desired soup consistency.

7. Add salt and pepper, to taste.

8. Serve warm.

COOKING TIP

Working with zucchini can be difficult due to its high water content. Do not skip towel drying the zucchini.

If you wanted to add another vegetable to this soup, add sautéed broccoli to the food processor with the zucchini. It will make a thicker soup, so you may want to increase the broth.

If you would like more onion or garlic once blended, add some garlic powder and/or onion powder to the processor as well. Remember that one garlic clove equals ⅛ tsp of garlic powder, and one medium chopped onion equals 1 T onion powder. Your best bet is to put in a little at a time, and taste test. If you put in too much, there is no going back.

NUTRITION NOTE

Zucchini is a good source of vitamin C, with over 50 percent of the recommended daily value in one medium zucchini. It also has a good amount of vitamin B6 (pyridoxine). Pyridoxine is needed to maintain the health of nerves, skin, and red blood cells.

Gazpacho Salad

Prep Time: 15 minutes

INGREDIENTS

1 pint heirloom cherry or grape tomatoes, cut in half

1 medium-sized cucumber, cut into bite-sized pieces

1 red bell pepper, cut into bite-sized pieces

1 T olive oil

2 T white or regular balsamic vinegar

1 tsp oregano

1 tsp dried basil

Salt and pepper, to taste

DIRECTIONS

1. Combine all ingredients, and mix thoroughly. Then chill in refrigerator, and serve.

Guacamole

Prep Time: 15 minutes

INGREDIENTS

3 avocados

2 plum tomatoes, diced

2 garlic cloves, minced

1 tsp onion powder

Salt and pepper, to taste

2 tsp lime zest (I actually use 2 drops of lime essential oil)

Squeeze of lime juice, to taste (optional, if you like more acidity)

DIRECTIONS

1. Wash and cut avocados in half. Scoop out flesh and put into a medium-sized bowl. Mash.

2. Add all ingredients, and mix to combine.

3. Cover and refrigerate until serving.

NUTRITION NOTE

Not all essential oils are meant for ingestion. If you choose to use essential oils when cooking or baking, make sure you have pure oils. A little goes a long way.

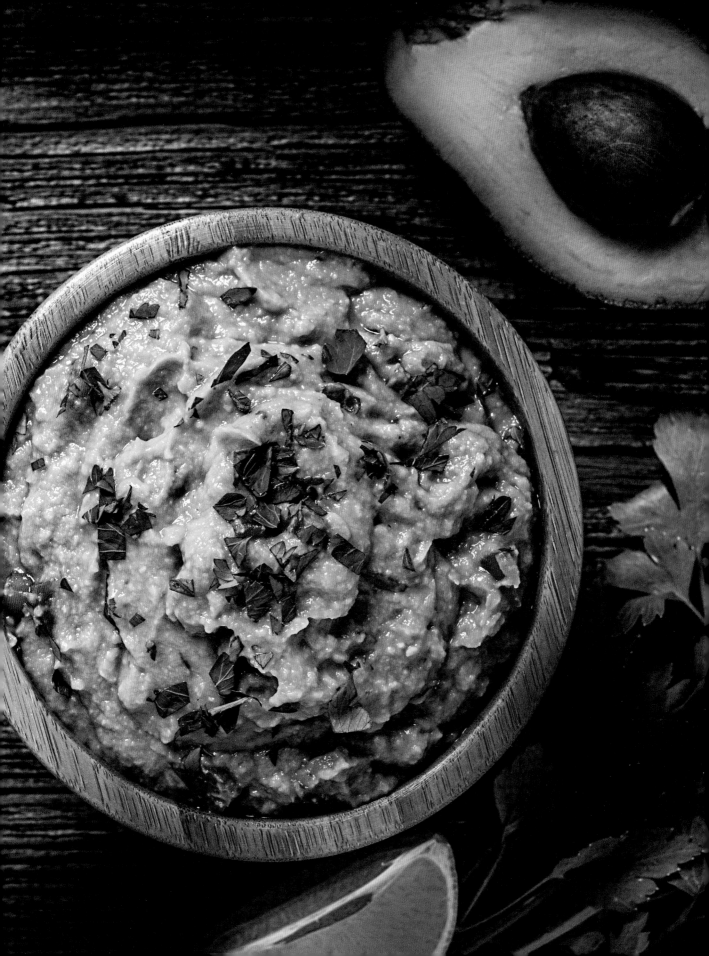

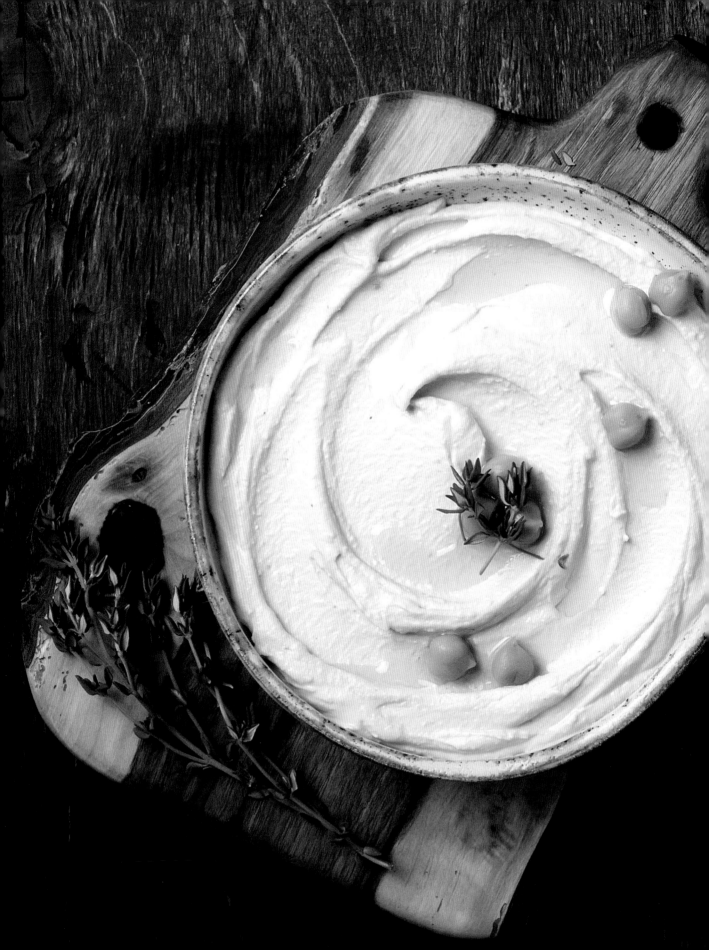

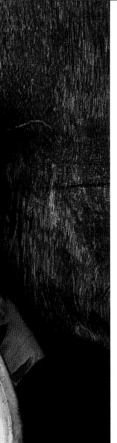

Tahini-Free Hummus

Prep Time: 15 minutes

INGREDIENTS

1 15-oz can of chickpeas

3 large garlic cloves,
    peeled and whole

⅓ cup water

1½ T olive oil

1 T fresh-squeezed lemon

¼ tsp cumin

Salt, to taste

DIRECTIONS

1. Drain and rinse chickpeas.

2. Put chickpeas in a bowl of warm
    water for 1–2 minutes, and peel the
    skins off. They should come off easily.

3. While you are soaking the chickpeas,
    put the garlic cloves into boiling
    water for 1 minute. This will give the
    garlic a milder flavor, and it won't
    overpower the other ingredients.

4. Put all ingredients into a food
    processor. Blend until smooth.

5. Taste. Adjust salt, as desired. Add a
    bit more lemon or cumin if you want.

COOKING TIP
It is a little time-consuming to take off the chickpea skin, but it is time
well invested. The texture of the hummus will be a lot smoother
and creamier.

NUTRITION NOTE
Chickpeas, also known as garbanzo beans, are rich in protein and fiber.
They also have a low glycemic index, which means your body absorbs
and digests them slowly. Chickpeas contain calcium and magnesium,
which promote bone health.

Zucchini Bites

Makes about 12 bites.
Prep Time: 15 minutes
Cook Time: 40 minutes

INGREDIENTS

2 tsp oil, separated (1 tsp for sautéing; 1 tsp for baking sheet)

2 garlic cloves, minced

2 medium zucchinis, grated

Salt and pepper, to taste

½ cup italian breadcrumbs*

¼ cup grated cheese*

1 tsp garlic powder

1 tsp onion powder

DIRECTIONS

1. Preheat oven to 375 degrees.

2. Heat oil in pan at low/medium heat, and sauté garlic about 2 minutes.

3. Add grated zucchini to pan, and combine with garlic. Season with salt and pepper, cover, and cook on low/medium heat about 7 minutes, until soft.

4. Transfer to a colander to remove excess water.

5. In a large bowl, combine zucchini, breadcrumbs,* cheese,* garlic powder, and onion powder.

6. Form into balls (about 1.5 inches around), and place on aluminum foil-lined baking sheet that has been coated with a thin layer of oil or cooking spray.

7. Bake 25 minutes.

COOKING TIP

If your zucchinis are small, decrease the quantity of breadcrumbs to ⅓ cup. If they are very large, then increase your breadcrumbs to ⅔ cup, or use just one zucchini.

*See the appendix for allergy-friendly alternatives.

Mains

broke this chapter down into nonvegetarian and vegetarian dishes. For the nonvegetarian recipes, I focused on poultry rather than red meat. Poultry has less saturated fat than red meat, and too much red meat can lead to elevated cholesterol levels. You can substitute red meat if you prefer, but do so in moderation. Plant-based diets are all the rage right now and for good reason, but as an allergy family, vegetarian sources of protein can be problematic since soy, eggs, nuts, dairy, and sesame are all top allergens. This is why I have included a large variety of nonvegetarian main meal options. Protein is important for proper growth and development, so if your child has multiple food allergies, as ours does, a vegetarian option may not be possible every day. Most of these recipes serve four, specifically two adults and two children, with potential for leftovers in some recipes like the pasta dishes.

Chicken is so versatile that it's no wonder it is the most loved nonvegetarian protein. When cooking chicken, stick to baking, broiling, or sautéing with a little oil and/or low sodium chicken broth. Frying chicken increases the calories and fat grams. It is not a good option nutrition-wise. Try to eat white meat the majority of the time, with little splurges of dark, and always remove the skin.

Families constantly ask me for a variety of chicken recipes so that their dinner options don't become too repetitive. This set of recipes will give you a number of healthy and tasty options for all that chicken you buy. Our family's favorite chicken recipe may surprise you. It's the chicken nugget recipe. Chicken nuggets are simple, but the way we cook them makes them crisp on the outside and juicy in the middle, plus they are gluten-free. There are never any leftovers when chicken nuggets are on the menu! My children have never eaten fast food because of their allergies and because it is not a healthy choice. I'm sure if we didn't have food allergies, we would have at least tried chicken nuggets from a fast-food chain, but I know my children would still be asking for Mom's version, hands down.

I also wanted to try to make a favorite of my husband's healthier and allergy-friendly, so that is how I came up with the chicken parm sliders. This is an easy recipe that uses ground chicken and tons of spices and sauce. It is delicious, and it really tastes like chicken parm without being fried.

For nights when you have very little time, try the garlic chicken thighs. The prep is minimal, but the taste is bold. If you love garlic, this recipe is for you.

We have a vegetable garden where we grow a number of things, including basil. Basil is probably my favorite herb, so I had to create a recipe that included it. That's how chicken with balsamic tomatoes and basil came about. If you already have a garden or are thinking of starting one, you will see that with many of these recipes, you can simply go to your garden and pick a lot of the ingredients right from there.

For the turkey recipes, opt for a lean ground turkey, such as 93/7. This means it is 93 percent lean meat and 7 percent fat. Lean beef is still an acceptable substitute for the lean ground turkey in any of these recipes. If you choose to use ground beef, go for 95 percent lean and 5 percent fat. The key to cooking with ground turkey is the herbs and spices. Turkey isn't very flavorful on its own, so what you add to it is important. One of the first recipes I ever created with the help of my mom is the sweet potato turkey loaf. I did not love meatloaf as a child, so I didn't know if we could create something that the whole family would enjoy, but we did it. The sweet potato adds sweetness to the ground turkey, which is delicious and acts as a binder, so you don't need the egg. Whenever we don't know what to make for dinner and we have ground turkey in the house, this is our go-to. We always seem to have a sweet potato lying around, since this has always been a favorite of our daughter's. I bet this is why we thought to incorporate it into the loaf when she was a baby. She was hooked after her first bite. This is another recipe where there are usually no leftovers.

I created two different meatball recipes because meatballs are a common food that children enjoy. One is a baked meatball recipe, and the other is a slow cooker recipe. The slow cooker recipe is one of the original recipes I created when we were first diagnosed with food allergies. Putting the meatballs in the slow cooker makes it an easy recipe for busy parents, and even without the egg, the meatballs come out tender due to the slow-cooking process.

This chapter also has a couple of nonvegetarian pasta recipes. My husband created Dad's Pasta Dish one day when he experimented with chicken and tons of veggies. The pasta "carbonara" recipe is a healthy take on a traditional favorite. It is simple to create and, of course, does not contain eggs. The triple-B mac and cheese contains turkey bacon, which I think my children would eat every day if I let them. The turkey bacon is delicious, and the nutrition from the butternut squash and broccoli make this dish a true winner in my book.

Nonvegetarian

Baked Chicken Cutlets

Prep Time: 10 minutes
Cook Time: 25 minutes

INGREDIENTS

3 boneless, skinless, chicken breasts

¼ cup italian breadcrumbs*

¼ cup grated cheese*

1 tsp garlic powder

1 tsp onion powder

½ tsp oregano

Salt, to taste

Milk or milk substitute for dipping*

DIRECTIONS

1. Preheat oven to 400 degrees.

2. Wrap breasts in plastic wrap, and pound until somewhat thin.

3. In a small bowl, mix breadcrumbs,* grated cheese,* garlic powder, onion powder, oregano, and salt.

4. Place chicken in a bowl, and coat with milk or milk substitute.*

5. Dip chicken into seasonings, covering all sides of the chicken.

6. Put chicken on an aluminum-foil-lined baking sheet.

7. Bake 25 minutes or until cooked through. Chicken is done when there is no longer any pink inside and it reaches an internal temperature of 165 degrees.

NUTRITION NOTE

Our family loves to make parsnip "fries" when we have chicken cutlets. Make them exactly like you would make sweet potato fries (recipe in vegetarian section). Parsnips are a root vegetable with a sweet taste, like carrots. Parsnips are a great source of vitamin C, vitamin K, and folate as well as fiber. You get 7 grams of fiber in one cup of parsnips.

*See the appendix for allergy-friendly alternatives.

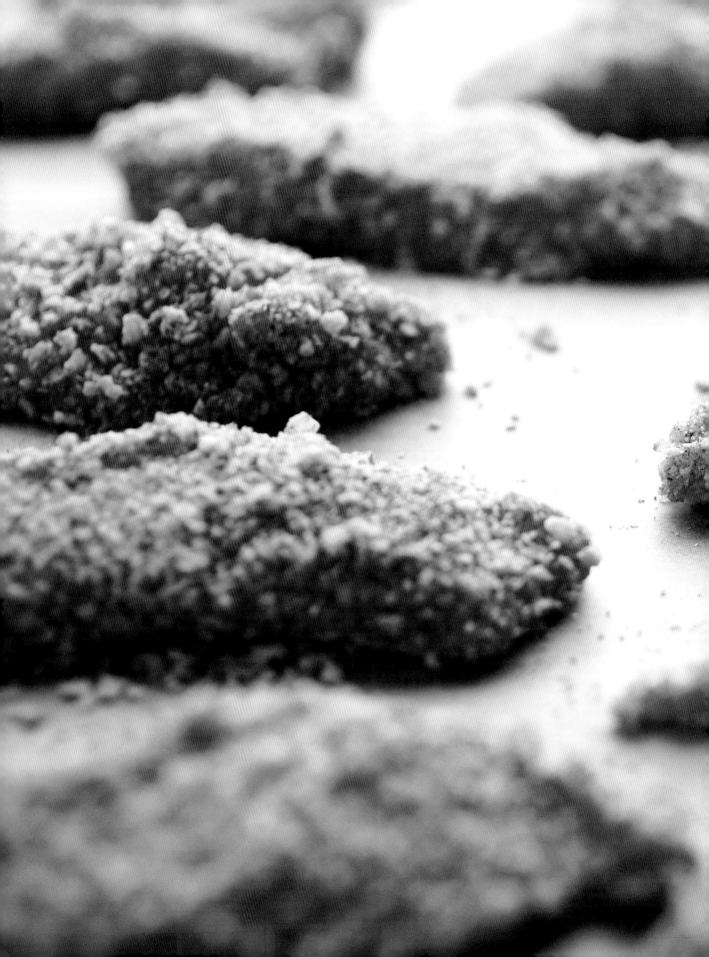

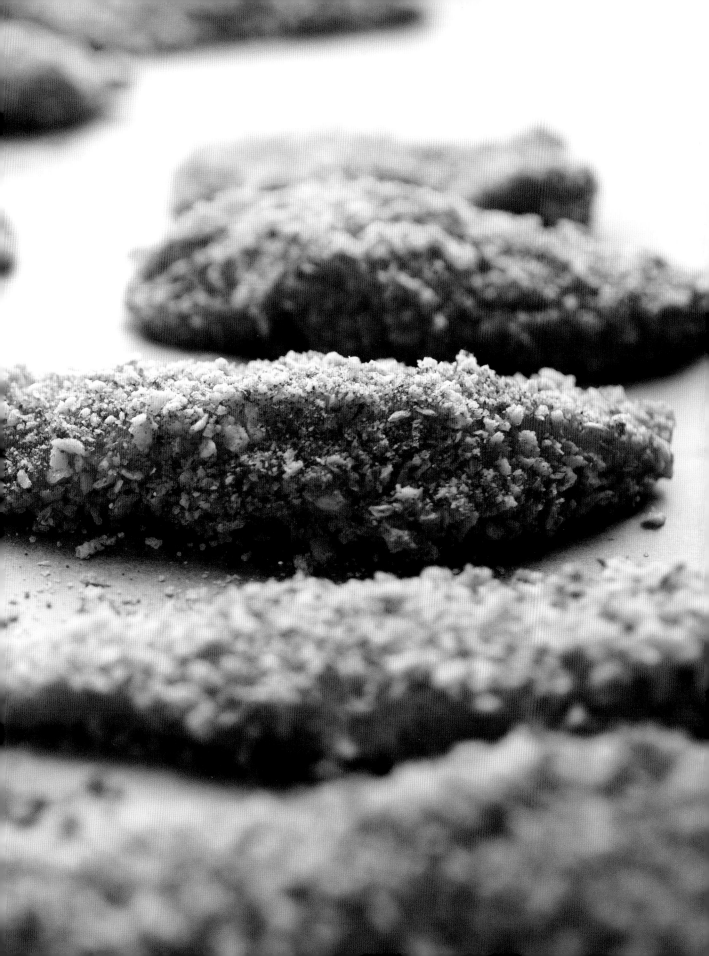

Chicken and Artichoke Orzo

Prep Time: 5 minutes
Cook Time: 25 minutes

INGREDIENTS

1½ cups uncooked gluten-free orzo*

1 T olive oil

2 garlic cloves, minced

4 boneless, skinless, thin-sliced chicken breasts

Salt and pepper, to taste

1½ cups tomato sauce

1 can of artichoke hearts in water, drained and quartered

2 T balsamic vinegar

2 tsp oregano

1 tsp dried basil

¼ cup shredded cheddar cheese*

DIRECTIONS

1. Cook orzo* according to package directions.

2. In a large pan, heat 1 T of olive oil on low/medium heat, and sauté garlic for two minutes.

3. Place chicken breasts in the pan on low/medium heat, and season with salt and pepper. Cover.

4. Cook chicken until outside is golden brown and middle is no longer pink. Cooking times vary depending on thickness of breast, about seven minutes per side or until internal temperature reaches 165 degrees.

5. When chicken is cooking, combine tomato sauce, artichokes, vinegar, oregano, and basil in a bowl and set aside.

6. Transfer chicken to a plate when completely cooked.

7. Turn heat down to low, and pour sauce into pan used to cook chicken.

8. Add cooked orzo* and cheese.* Mix until blended.

9. Slice chicken into bite-sized pieces, and add to the pan. Combine.

COOKING TIP

Our family also likes to separate the components and build the meal on our plates. For example, rather than combining the sauce, chicken, orzo, and cheese, we put the plain orzo on our plates, top it with artichoke tomato sauce and sliced chicken, and sprinkle shredded cheese. This way, if someone doesn't want sauce or any other ingredient that day, which happens a lot with children, they can make that decision. This is a good tip when it comes to feeding young children. Give them choices, and separate the ingredients. A lot of children do not like meals that mix several ingredients together.

NUTRITION NOTE

We like this dish with gluten-free orzo, but you can use any gluten-free pasta.

*See the appendix for allergy-friendly alternatives.

Baked Chicken Nuggets

Prep Time: 10 minutes
Cook Time: 25 minutes

INGREDIENTS

⅓ cup italian breadcrumbs*

⅛ cup grated cheese*

1 tsp garlic powder

1 tsp onion powder

2–3 boneless, skinless, chicken breasts

¼ cup melted butter or butter substitute*

DIRECTIONS

1. Preheat oven to 400 degrees.

2. Mix breadcrumbs,* grated cheese,* garlic powder, and onion powder in a bowl.

3. Cut chicken into nugget-sized pieces.

4. Dip them into melted butter,* and then dip them into the breadcrumb mixture.

5. Place on an aluminum foil-lined baking sheet.

6. Bake for 25 minutes at 400 degrees or until nuggets reach an internal temperature of 165 degrees.

COOKING TIP

You don't have to dip one nugget into the butter and breadcrumbs at a time. I usually grab a large handful to speed up the process.

NUTRITION NOTE

These nuggets are delicious and, with just six ingredients, are much healthier than fast-food nuggets. My family eats them so quickly that I barely have time to transfer them from the baking sheet to a plate.

*See the appendix for allergy-friendly alternatives.

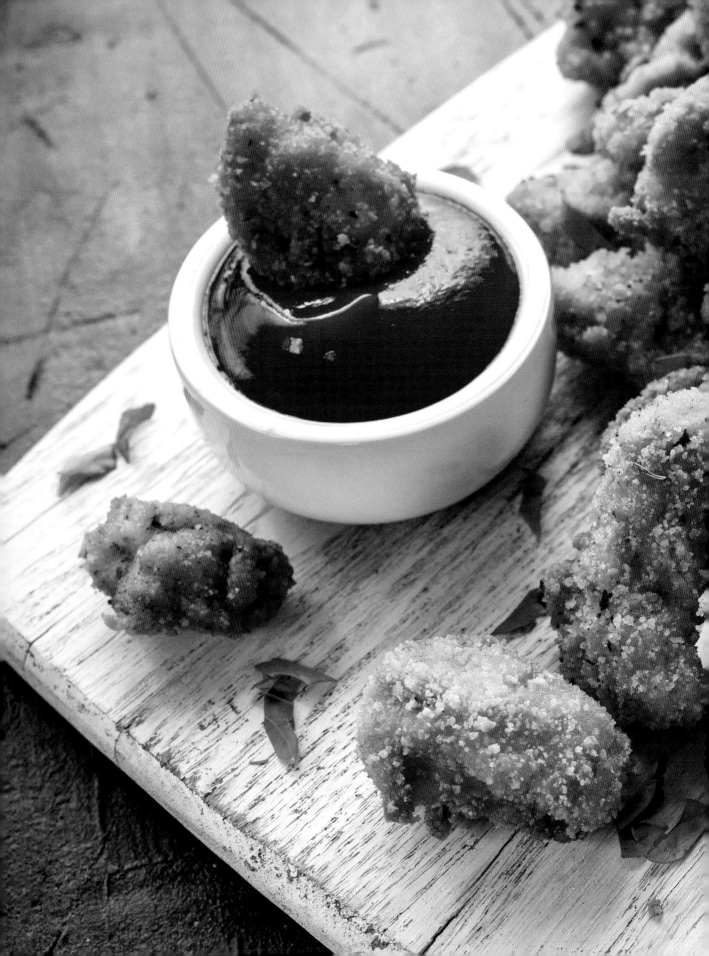

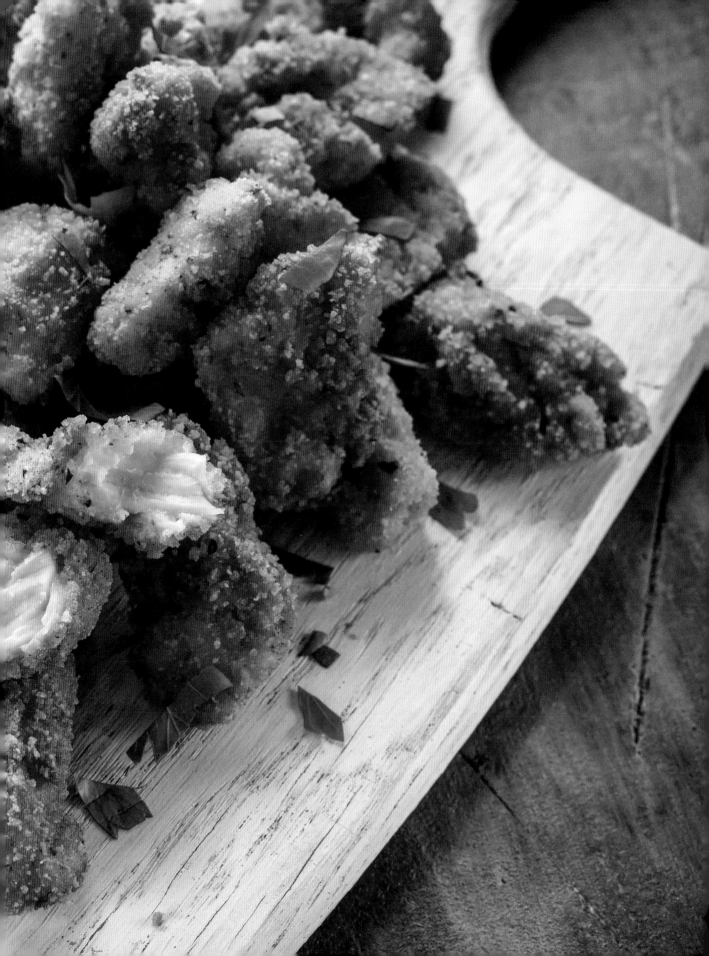

Chicken with Corn and Roasted Tomatoes

Prep Time: 10 minutes
Cook Time: 25 minutes

INGREDIENTS

Pint of grape or cherry tomatoes, cut lengthwise

2 T oil (separated)

2 garlic cloves, minced

3 T fresh basil leaves, chopped

3–4 boneless, skinless, thin-sliced chicken breasts

½ tsp garlic powder

½ tsp oregano

1 bag of frozen corn (8–10 oz bag) or 4 fresh cobs of corn

6 cups raw baby spinach

Salt, to taste

DIRECTIONS

1. Preheat oven to 400 degrees.

2. Place tomatoes on an aluminum foil-lined baking sheet. Drizzle with 1 T olive oil and top with minced garlic and basil.

3. Wrap the foil around the tomato mixture, sealing tightly to keep tomato juices inside.

4. Place chicken breasts on a separate lined baking sheet, and sprinkle with salt, garlic powder, and oregano.

5. Put chicken and tomato mixture into oven for 20–25 minutes at 400 degrees or until chicken reaches an internal temperature of 165 degrees.

6. If using frozen corn, cook to package directions. If using corn on the cob, boil for about 5–7 minutes, and cut kernels off of the cob.

7. Sauté spinach in 1 T of oil. Add salt, to taste.

8. When chicken is cooked through and tomatoes are roasted, remove from oven.

COOKING TIP

When serving, you always have a choice. Plate the corn, tomatoes, and spinach separately and add sliced chicken on top, or cut the chicken into bite-sized pieces and combine with corn, tomatoes, and spinach. Everyone in our home does it a little differently. When you have children, you don't necessarily have to cook multiple different meals. How you serve the meal may be what interests them in trying it. It's all about giving children a little bit of choice but not so much as to overwhelm them.

Chicken with Balsamic Tomatoes and Basil

Prep Time: 10 minutes
Cook Time: 25 minutes

INGREDIENTS

1 lb boneless, skinless, thin-sliced
   chicken breasts

Salt and pepper, to taste

1 T oil

1 large garlic clove, minced

¼ cup balsamic vinegar

1 pint grape tomatoes, cut in half lengthwise

¼ cup fresh basil, chopped

DIRECTIONS

1. Preheat oven to 425 degrees.

2. Sprinkle salt and pepper on chicken, and bake for 20–25 minutes or until internal temperature reaches 165 degrees.

3. As chicken is cooking, heat oil in a medium-sized pan over low/medium heat.

4. Add garlic and sauté until fragrant, 1–2 minutes.

5. Add vinegar, and reduce for 3–4 minutes.

6. Add tomatoes. Cover and let simmer about 5 minutes or until soft, stirring occasionally.

7. When chicken is cooked, place in pan with tomato mixture and cover with the sauce. Add basil.

NUTRITION NOTE

Not only is basil delicious, it is also very good for you. Those in Asia, where basil originated, held basil as a sacred and noble herb. The word *basil* means *royal*. Basil contains many vitamins and minerals, as well as antioxidants. The antioxidants mostly disappear during the drying process, so opt for fresh basil whenever possible.

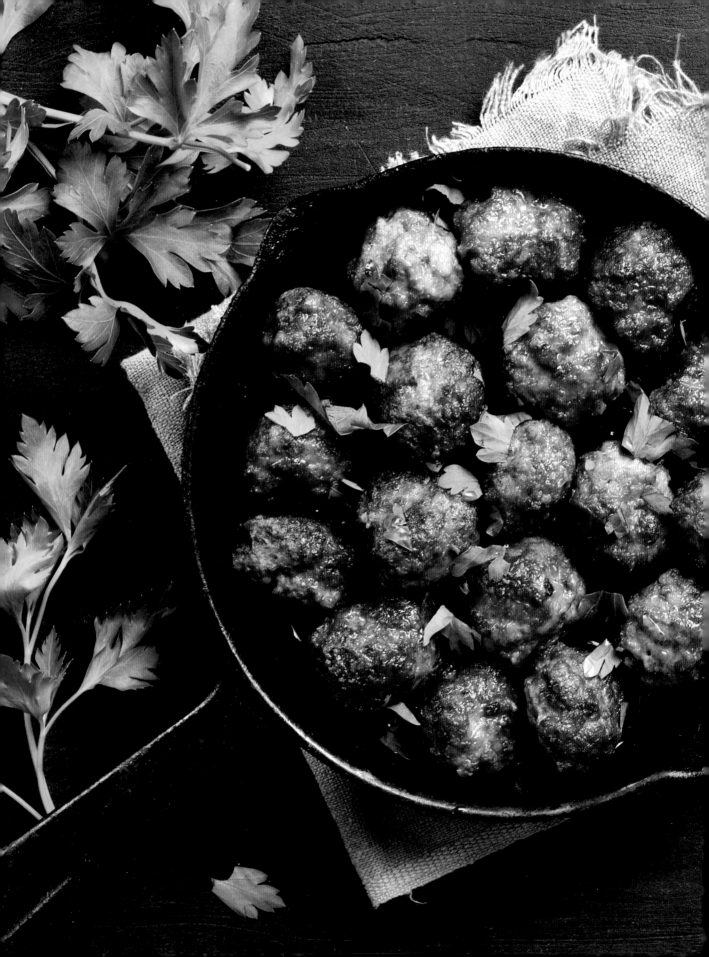

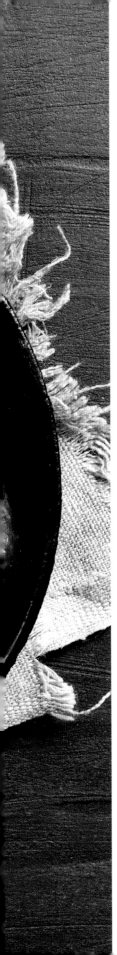

Baked Turkey Meatballs

Makes 18 meatballs.
Prep Time: 10 minutes
Cook Time: 25 minutes

INGREDIENTS

1 lb lean ground turkey

⅓ cup italian breadcrumbs*

½ tsp of each seasoning
(garlic powder, onion powder,
oregano, dried basil)

¼ cup grated cheese*

DIRECTIONS

1. Preheat oven to 425 degrees.

2. Mix all ingredients in a medium-sized mixing bowl.

3. Form meatballs (about 2 inches in diameter), place on lined baking sheet or cast-iron skillet, and bake for 25 minutes.

COOKING TIP

Who wants meatballs without pasta? A great alternative to pasta is spaghetti squash. Cut the squash in half, and scoop out the seeds. Drizzle with oil. Place the cut side down on a baking sheet and roast for about 40 minutes. You can also try zoodles (zucchini noodles), if you prefer.

*See the appendix for allergy-friendly alternatives.

Garlic Chicken Thighs

Prep Time: 5 minutes
Cook Time: 30 minutes

INGREDIENTS

4–6 boneless, skinless, chicken thighs

2 T oil

4 garlic cloves, minced

2 T lemon zest

Drizzle of honey

DIRECTIONS

1. Preheat oven to 425 degrees.

2. Place chicken thighs on a baking sheet lined with aluminum foil.

3. In a small bowl, combine oil, garlic, and lemon zest. Pour mixture over each thigh.

4. Drizzle each thigh with a little honey for a touch of sweetness.

5. Bake 30 minutes or until chicken reaches an internal temperature of 165 degrees.

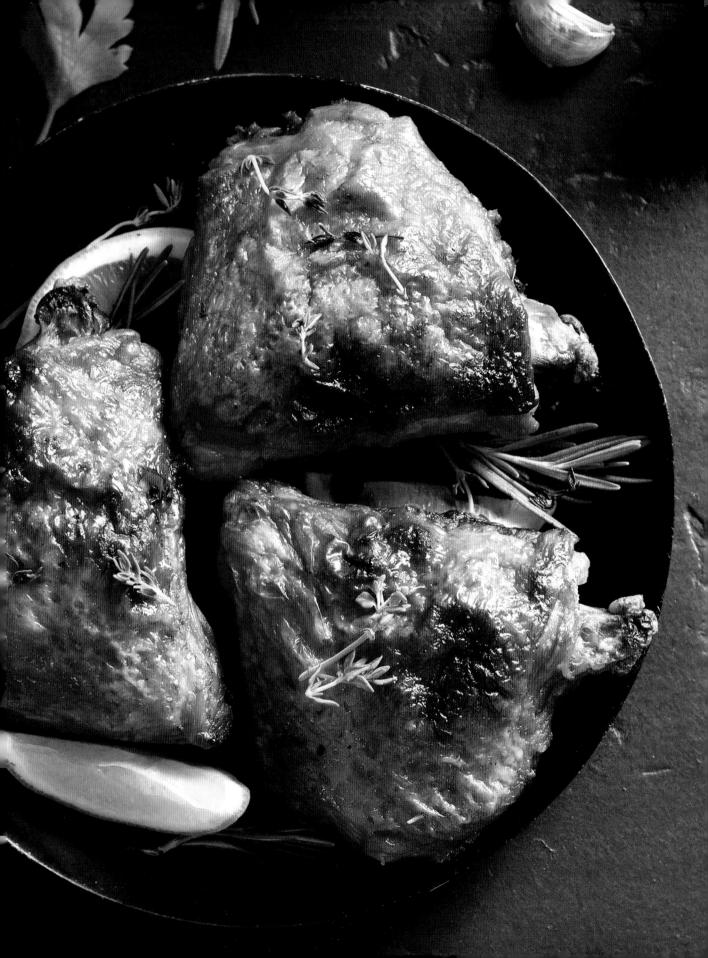

Crockpot Turkey Meatballs and Carrots

Makes about 12 meatballs.

Prep Time: 10 minutes

Cook Time: 4–6 hours

INGREDIENTS

Bag of baby carrots or a bag of fresh carrots cut into baby size

1 lb lean ground turkey

⅓ cup of italian breadcrumbs*

1 tsp garlic powder

1 tsp onion powder

1 tsp oregano

1 15-oz can of tomato sauce

DIRECTIONS

1. Place carrots at the bottom of slow cooker.

2. In a large bowl, mix together ground turkey, breadcrumbs,* garlic powder, onion powder, and oregano.

3. Shape into medium-sized meatballs, and place on top of the carrots.

4. Pour the entire can of sauce on top of the carrots and meatballs.

5. Cook for 4 hours on high or 6 hours on low.

NUTRITION NOTE

Carrots are an excellent source of vitamin A in the form of beta-carotene. They are also a good source of several B vitamins, as well as vitamin K and potassium.

*See the appendix for allergy-friendly alternatives.

Ground Turkey and Veggie Bowl

Prep Time: 15 minutes
Cook Time: 20 minutes

INGREDIENTS

1 T oil

½ small yellow onion, diced

3 garlic cloves, minced

1 lb lean ground turkey

1 large zucchini, chopped into bite-sized pieces

1 15-oz can of diced tomatoes

1 T tomato paste

1 tsp dried oregano

Salt and pepper, to taste

¼ avocado, sliced, to top

DIRECTIONS

1. Heat medium-sized pan over low/medium heat, and add olive oil.

2. Sauté onion and garlic for 2 minutes until fragrant.

3. Turn heat to medium, add turkey, and cook about 5–7 minutes. Chop up the turkey during this time.

4. Add zucchini, stir, and cover. Cook another 3–5 minutes.

5. Add diced tomatoes, tomato paste, and oregano. Stir together.

6. Reduce heat to low, and simmer 5 minutes or until turkey is completely cooked through and an internal temperature of 165 degrees is reached.

7. Add salt and pepper, to taste.

8. Top with avocado when serving.

NUTRITION NOTE

If you wanted to add a starch to this recipe, scoop it over gluten-free pasta, rice, or any other starch you like.

Pasta "Carbonara"

Prep Time: 5 minutes
Cook Time: 10 minutes

INGREDIENTS

1 lb dried pasta*

Bag of frozen peas (about 2 cups)

¾ cup low fat milk or milk substitute*

1 tsp onion powder

1 cup shredded cheese*

4 slices deli ham or fresh ham
    cut into 1-inch squares

DIRECTIONS

1. In a large pot, cook pasta* to package directions. Add frozen peas near the end of cooking.

2. In another pot, add milk,* onion powder, and shredded cheese.* Whisk well, and bring to a simmer.

3. As soon as cheese* melts, reduce heat to low, and add to drained peas and rigatoni. Add ham, and gently combine.

COOKING TIP

This sauce is very light. If you prefer a thicker sauce, you can make a roux first, and then add the liquid and cheese. To make a roux:

1. Melt 2 T butter or butter substitute* in a saucepan over low/medium heat.

2. Add 2 T flour (rice flour works nicely), and whisk into the butter* until combined.

3. Slowly add about 1 cup of milk or milk substitute,* and mix until smooth and thickened. Turn off heat.

4. Stir in cheese* until combined.

*See the appendix for allergy-friendly alternatives.

Dad's Pasta Dish

Prep Time: 15 minutes
Cook Time: 30 minutes

INGREDIENTS

1 lb penne pasta*

2–3 boneless, skinless, thin-sliced chicken breasts

Seasoning: ½ teaspoon each of onion powder, garlic powder, and oregano

1 head of broccoli, chopped

2 T of oil, separated (1 T for roasting broccoli, 1 T for sautéing artichokes)

1 garlic clove, minced

1 can artichoke hearts in water, chopped

1 package of frozen spinach or 6 cups fresh baby spinach

Salt and pepper, to taste

Drizzle of olive oil and sprinkle of grated cheese* before serving

DIRECTIONS

1. Preheat oven to 400 degrees.

2. Cook pasta* to package directions.

3. While pasta* is cooking, season chicken with onion powder, garlic powder, and oregano. Put on an aluminum foil-lined baking sheet.

4. Spread broccoli florets on a separate baking sheet, drizzle with oil, and season with salt.

5. Put both chicken and broccoli in the oven for 25 minutes at 400 degrees or until internal temperature of chicken is 165 degrees and the broccoli is tender.

6. While the chicken and broccoli are in the oven, heat oil in a large pan or skillet over low/medium heat.

7. Sauté garlic in oil until fragrant (1–2 minutes). Add artichoke hearts, and turn heat down to low.

8. Cook frozen spinach to package directions, season with salt and pepper. If using fresh spinach, sauté with artichokes and garlic.

9. When chicken is done, cut into bite-sized pieces, and add to artichokes, along with roasted broccoli. Add pasta* and spinach to the pan. Combine.

10. Drizzle olive oil on top and sprinkle with grated cheese,* to taste.

NUTRITION NOTE

We have made this recipe with all sorts of vegetables, including peppers, zucchini, and peas. Choose your favorite, and switch it up each time to get different vitamins in every meal. My husband created this dish one day when we had no idea what to make for dinner. He combined tons of veggies, chicken, and spices, and the end result became one of my daughter's favorite meals. The moral of the story is, don't be afraid to experiment in the kitchen.

*See the appendix for allergy-friendly alternatives.

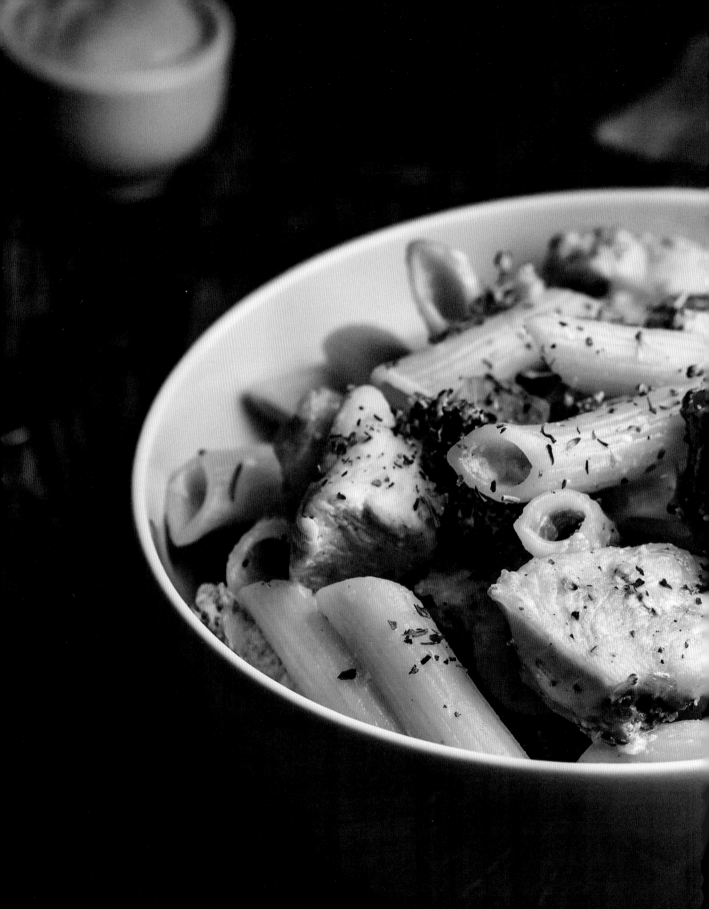

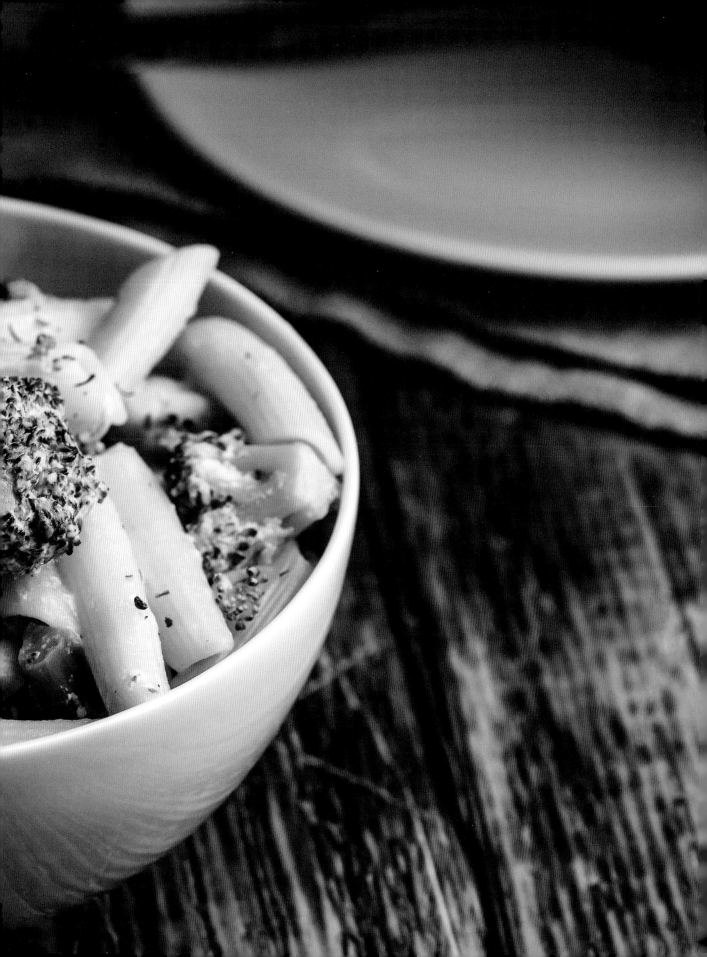

Parmesan-Style Chicken Burger

Makes 6 burgers.
Prep Time: 5 minutes
Cook Time: 15 minutes

INGREDIENTS

2 tsp oil (split 1 tsp and 1 tsp)

2 garlic cloves, minced

1 lb ground chicken

¾ cup tomato sauce

¼ cup grated cheese*

1 tsp onion powder

1 tsp oregano

DIRECTIONS

1. Heat medium-sized pan over low heat. Add 1 tsp oil to pan.

2. Sauté garlic for 2 minutes or until fragrant. Place sautéed garlic in a large bowl.

3. Add ground chicken, tomato sauce, cheese,* onion powder, and oregano to the bowl with the garlic. Combine well.

4. Shape into 6 slider patties. I use a large spoon to scoop out the mixture and shape into burgers on the pan.

5. Using the same pan, heat 1 tsp oil on low/medium heat, and add chicken burgers. Cover and cook 4–5 minutes per side, or until an internal temperature of 165 degrees is reached.

COOKING TIP
Before you cook the sliders, the ground chicken mixture may seem too wet, but once you cook them, they will be perfect. The added tomato sauce gives much-needed moisture to the lean ground chicken.

NUTRITION NOTE
Eat the chicken burgers on buns, on a plate alongside a vegetable, or added to a large salad for a low-carb option.

*See the appendix for allergy-friendly alternatives.

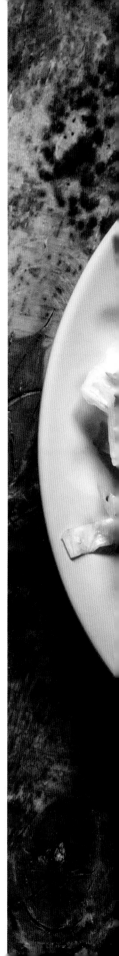

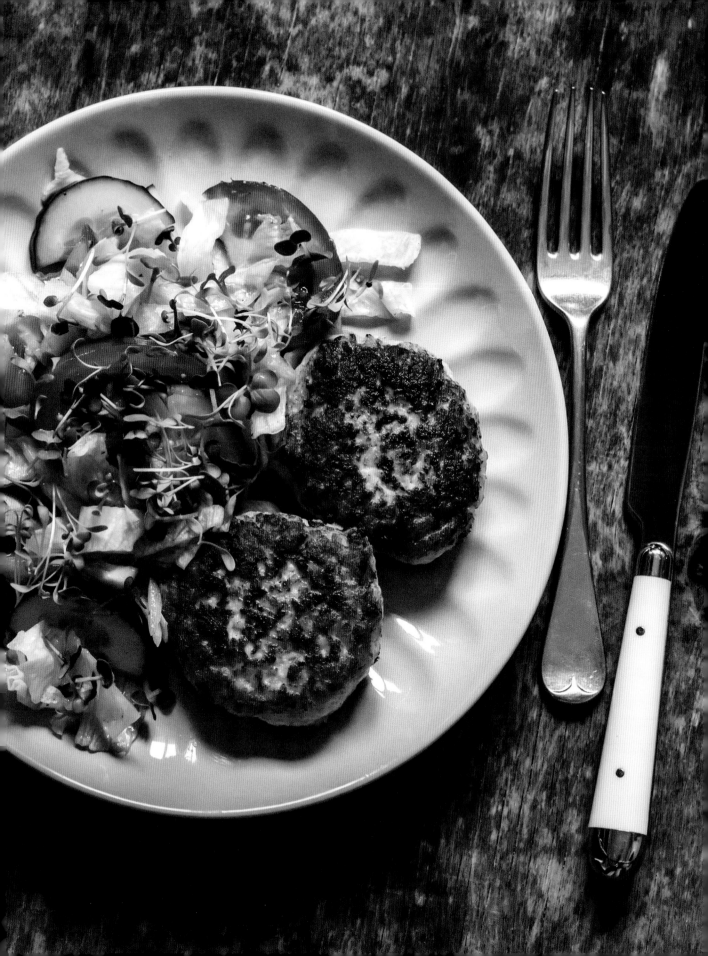

Triple-B Mac and Cheese

Prep Time: 15 minutes (longer if you are peeling and cubing the butternut squash yourself)
Cook Time: 35 minutes

INGREDIENTS

5 slices turkey bacon

1 T oil

3 garlic cloves, minced

2¼ cups unsalted chicken stock

1¼ cups milk or milk substitute*

Butternut squash, peeled and cubed into bite-sized pieces

½ lb uncooked elbow macaroni*

Bag of frozen broccoli florets

1 cup shredded cheese*

DIRECTIONS

1. Cook bacon in a large deep skillet until crispy, and set aside on a paper towel.

2. Turn heat to low/medium heat, and add 1 T of olive oil to bacon skillet.

3. Sauté garlic 2 minutes.

4. Add stock, milk,* and squash to pan. Bring to a boil. Stir occasionally.

5. Add uncooked pasta* and cover. Reduce heat to low and simmer for about 6 minutes, stirring occasionally.

6. Add broccoli. Cover and cook for an additional 3–5 minutes, or until pasta is al dente and sauce is thickened.

7. Remove skillet from heat, and stir in cheese* until melted. Crumble bacon on top.

COOKING TIP
Poke holes in your butternut squash and microwave on high for five minutes so it is easier to peel and cube, or buy already peeled and cubed squash at the grocery store.

NUTRITION NOTE
Butternut squash is a great fall vegetable. It is versatile and packed with vitamins A and C and potassium.

*See the appendix for allergy-friendly alternatives.

Sheet Pan Chicken and Asparagus

Prep Time: 10 minutes
Cook Time: 25 minutes

INGREDIENTS

1 lb bundle of asparagus
   (20–30 standard-sized spears)

1 T oil

3 boneless, skinless, thin-cut
   chicken breasts

1 tsp garlic powder

1 tsp onion powder

Salt and pepper, to taste

DIRECTIONS

1. Preheat oven to 400 degrees.

2. Wash the asparagus, and cut into 3-inch pieces. Place in a bowl and coat with 1 T of oil and salt to taste.

3. Line a baking sheet with aluminum foil. Place chicken in the middle, surrounded by asparagus.

4. Sprinkle garlic powder, onion powder, salt, and pepper on each chicken breast.

5. Put chicken and asparagus into the oven and bake for about 25 minutes or until the internal temperature of the chicken reaches 165 degrees.

COOKING TIP

You can also use regular instead of thin-cut chicken breasts if you prefer, but the baking time will increase by about 5 minutes or so.

Also, if asparagus isn't your favorite vegetable, you can swap it for any vegetable that roasts well. Some of our favorites are roasted kale and brussel sprouts. When working with kale, wash the leaves, dry them off, and place them on a lined baking sheet. Drizzle with oil and salt and bake for 10–12 minutes at 400 degrees. If something is in the oven with the kale, it may take a bit longer. These kale chips are so delicious that your kids will actually ask to eat kale! For brussel sprouts, cut them lengthwise, and drizzle with oil and salt. Bake for 25 minutes at 400 degrees.

NUTRITION NOTE

Asparagus is an excellent source of vitamin K, an essential nutrient involved in blood clotting and bone health. In addition, asparagus is high in folate, a nutrient that is vital for a healthy pregnancy and many important processes in the body, including cell growth and DNA formation.

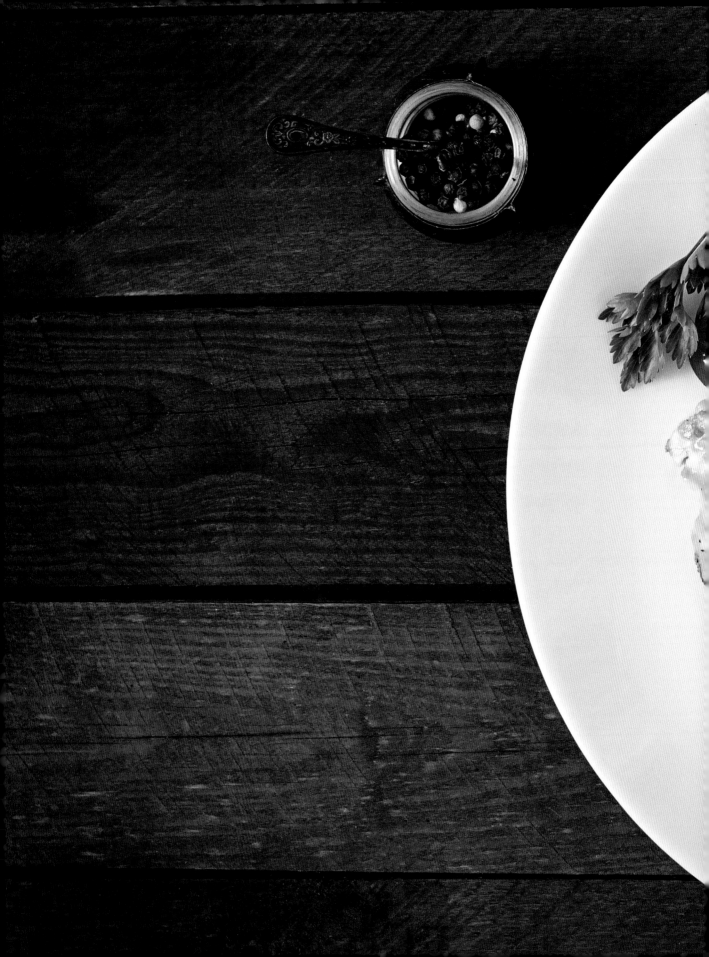

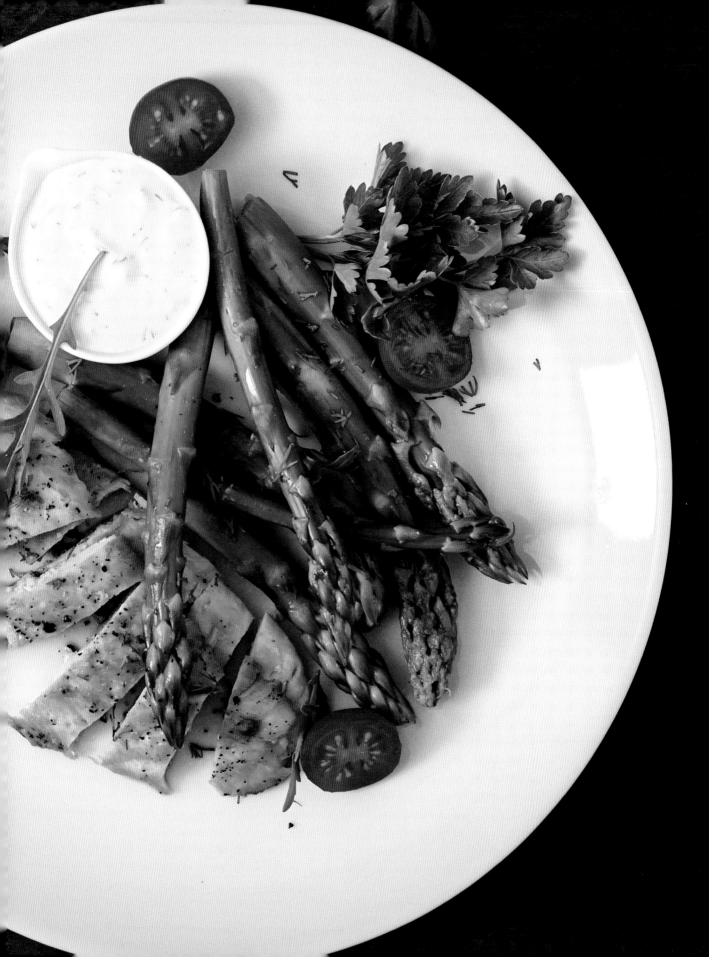

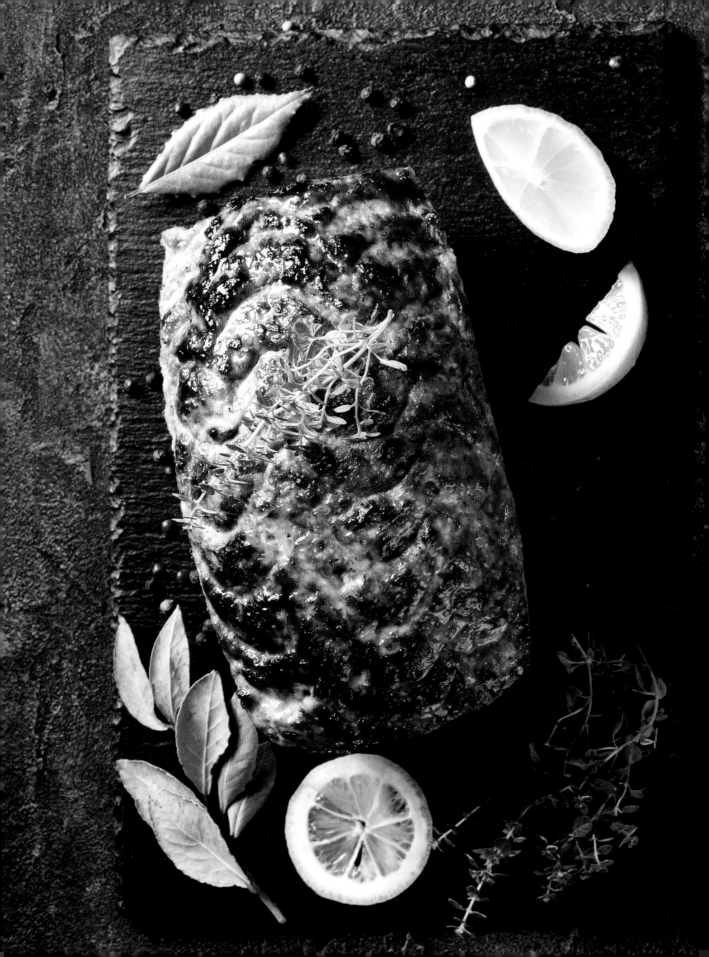

Sweet Potato Turkey Loaf

Prep Time: 15 minutes
Cook Time: 50 minutes

INGREDIENTS

1 medium to large sweet potato

1 lb lean ground turkey

2 T ketchup

¼ cup italian breadcrumbs*

1 tsp garlic powder

1 tsp onion powder

1 tsp oregano

¼ cup grated cheese*

DIRECTIONS

1. Preheat oven to 375 degrees.

2. Wash sweet potato, and poke it with a fork.

3. Microwave sweet potato on high for about 7 minutes, depending on size, and let cool. You know the sweet potato is done when you are able to easily scoop out the inside. It will be soft to the touch.

4. While waiting for sweet potato to cool place turkey, ketchup, breadcrumbs,* seasonings, and cheese* in a bowl.

5. When sweet potato is cooled, scoop out the inside from the skin, and add to the bowl.

6. Mix well, shape into a loaf, and place on a lined baking sheet or place into a nonstick loaf pan.

7. Bake for 50 minutes.

NUTRITION NOTE

Sweet potatoes are a rich source of fiber, as well as vitamins and minerals including iron, calcium, selenium, vitamin C, and most B vitamins. Sweet potatoes are also high in beta-carotene, which converts to vitamin A once you eat it.

For increased sweetness, add an additional swirl of ketchup on top before baking. Sometimes we write the children's initials on top with ketchup. Any way you can get kids involved with cooking, go for it.

*See the appendix for allergy-friendly alternatives.

Ginger-Baked Whole Chicken

Prep Time: 10 minutes
Cook Time: 1 hour and 10 minutes

INGREDIENTS

4–5 lb whole chicken

1 2-inch piece of peeled ginger, cut into thin slices

3 cloves of garlic, 1 peeled and sliced thin, 2 kept whole

1 T oil

1 tsp paprika

1 tsp cinnamon

1 tsp grated ginger (fresh)

DIRECTIONS

1. Preheat oven to 450 degrees.

2. Place chicken into a baking dish, breast side up.

3. Loosen the skin from the breast, and place the sliced ginger and sliced garlic under the skin.

4. Place the 2 whole garlic cloves inside the chicken.

5. Rub oil on the outside of the chicken. This will make the skin crispier.

6. Sprinkle paprika, cinnamon, and grated ginger onto the chicken, and rub all over.

7. Bake for 20 minutes at 450 degrees, and then an additional 50 minutes at 350 degrees or until internal temperature of chicken reaches 165 degrees and juices run clear. Use a meat thermometer for this step. Let the chicken rest 10 minutes before you slice into it.

COOKING TIP
Use leftover chicken for soup. The ginger gives it a nice flavor and is helpful in lessening cold symptoms.

NUTRITION NOTE
Ginger is known to have multiple benefits, including reducing nausea, pain, and inflammation. You can also add a sprinkle of turmeric for added health benefits.

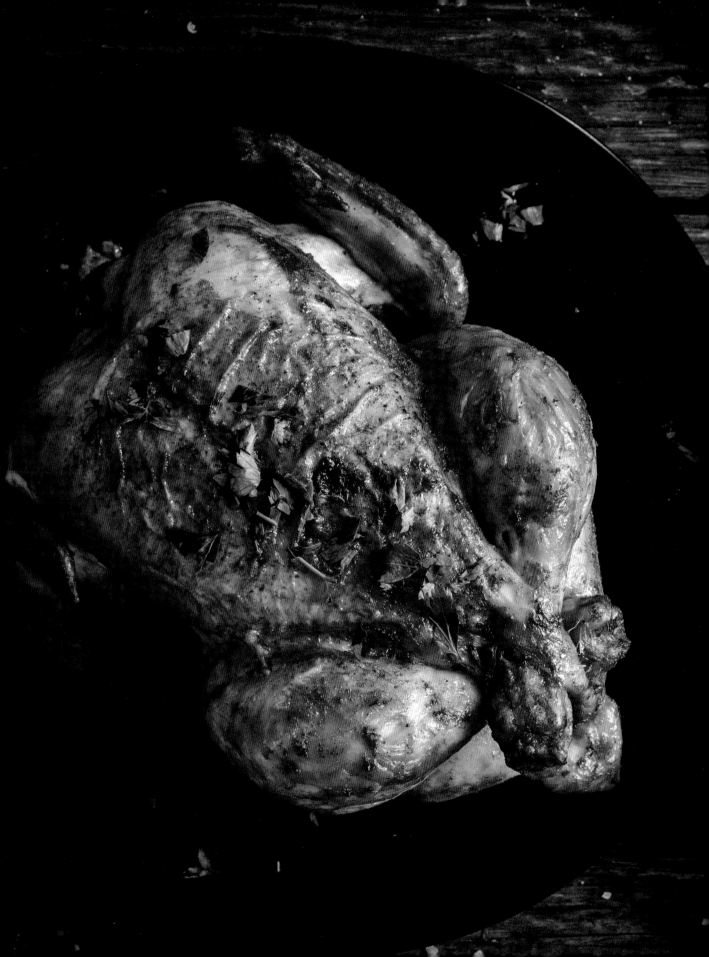

Turkey Burgers

Prep Time: 5 minutes
Cook Time: 20 minutes

INGREDIENTS

1 lb lean ground turkey

1 tsp onion powder

½ tsp pepper

1 T oil

1 large garlic clove, minced

Thinly sliced avocado, lettuce, tomato, and turkey bacon for topping

DIRECTIONS

1. In a medium-sized mixing bowl, add turkey, onion powder, and pepper. Set aside.

2. Heat oil in a pan over medium heat.

3. Add minced garlic and sauté for 1–2 minutes.

4. Put garlic into the turkey bowl.

5. Mix by hand to form into 4 patties.

6. Place patties in pan and cover. Cook for about 6 minutes. Flip, cover, and cook for another 6 minutes or until an internal temperature of 165 degrees is reached.

7. Put onto a gluten-free bun and add sliced avocado and other toppings, as listed.

Turkey Sloppy Joe

Prep Time: 10 minutes
Cook Time: 20 minutes

INGREDIENTS

1 T oil

2 garlic cloves, minced

1 lb lean ground turkey

1 tsp garlic powder

1 tsp onion powder

½ tsp chili powder

¼ tsp smoked paprika

1 large carrot, grated

1 green zucchini, grated

1 15-oz can of pure tomato sauce

¼ cup ketchup

1 T tomato paste

1 T red wine vinegar

1 avocado, sliced thin

DIRECTIONS

1. In a large pan, heat oil over low heat. Add minced garlic and sauté for 1 minute.

2. Add turkey and cook through (about 7 minutes). Chop it up with a spatula.

3. Add spices, carrots, and zucchini. Stir and simmer for 3 minutes. Make sure to mix all the seasonings in thoroughly.

4. Add can of tomato sauce, ketchup, tomato paste, and red wine vinegar. Stir and simmer for 5–7 minutes.

5. Serve by itself with sliced avocado on top or on a gluten-free hamburger bun or toasted English muffin.*

COOKING TIP

Adjust spices according to your family's spice tolerance. You may want to up the chili powder to 1 tsp if your family wants a little more kick.

*See the appendix for allergy-friendly alternatives.

Vegetarian

This section will give you some delicious vegetarian dishes to try. Aim to fill your family's diet with tons of vegetables and legumes. They have many nutrients that you can't get from any other foods. Try your best to incorporate vegetables into every meal, if possible, or at least one or two meals a day and snacks. The goal is a minimum of five servings of fruit and vegetables daily— specifically, two servings of fruit and three servings of vegetables. One serving is half a cup of any vegetables or roughly one cup of leafy greens or fruit. The research shows that eating this amount can lower your risk of heart disease, cancer, and respiratory disease. Keep trying to find ways to incorporate them into your diet in any way you can.

As a dietitian, I recommend a plant-based diet to my patients. This doesn't mean you need to be a strict vegetarian, but it does mean that vegetables are a large part of your diet and that not every meal needs to be centered around an animal protein. In our family, we probably eat poultry twice a week, fish once, and then the rest is vegetarian. Beans of all types and quinoa are our top two protein-rich foods that we use in a lot of our vegetarian meals. They also are not top allergens, so hopefully most families can enjoy these foods as well. The quinoa veggie bowl is one of my personal favorites. You can add any veggies you want, and the lemon garlic dressing enhances the flavor. If your children won't try quinoa, add this dressing to it, and they may surprise you. Our son did. The vegetarian tacos are great for kids because they get to take part in the preparation by choosing their own toppings. We lay a variety of toppings out, and they create their own personalized tacos.

I definitely couldn't leave out creating a veggie burger. Many veggie burgers have soy in them, so I was determined to create one without. This took a lot of trial and error, but when I finally got it, it worked well. It takes a bit more time to prepare, but if you want to create a soy-free veggie burger, try this recipe.

Pasta is also a go-to for a lot of families since it is quick and easy to make, but it may not contain much nutrients. The pasta recipes included in this section have vegetables added to them, and in one recipe they are even "hidden." There are many allergy-friendly options for pasta. These recipes are written so you can incorporate whatever variety of pasta is safe for your specific allergies. If you have a gluten allergy, please refer to the appendix for alternative brands to use. Whole-grain pasta or pasta made from legumes are better options than white pasta due to the increased fiber and protein. White or refined pasta is made by stripping the outer layers of the grain, which are packed with fiber, and grinding up only the inside portion of the grain. What remains has some nutrients, but many more are missing. If the first word on the ingredient label is *enriched*, your pasta is not made from a whole grain. Avoid the term *enriched*, and make sure the first ingredient includes *whole* or a legume.

Pasta is probably our daughter's favorite food to eat, so I knew I had to come up with some tasty, nutritious, and—of course—safe options for her and the rest of the family. I took every family's favorite recipes, such as lasagna and mac and cheese, and put a healthy twist to them, while keeping them free of the top nine allergens. I don't know about your family, but my kids would eat mac and cheese everyday if I let them. Out of all the pasta recipes, hidden-veggie mac and cheese is number one. When they were younger, they didn't even know it wasn't the traditional mac and cheese. As they got older, they saw me add the carrots and the butternut squash, so of course, they questioned me. We spoke about the benefits of these veggies, and I reminded them how delicious it was. My son is harder to please, and he gobbles it up, even after knowing there are vegetables in it.

Butternut Spinach Lasagna

Prep Time: 15 minutes
Cook Time: 1 hour and 5 minutes

INGREDIENTS

4 cups butternut squash, cut into small bite-sized pieces

Lasagna noodles (about 9)*

5 cups baby spinach

2 T oil (separated)

1 garlic clove, minced

1 15-oz can of tomato sauce

Seasoning: 1 tsp oregano,
    1 tsp garlic powder,
    1 tsp onion powder, and
    1 tsp dried basil

⅔ cup ricotta cheese
    (use about 3 oz of dairy-free shreds as a substitute)*

1 oz shredded mozzarella*

DIRECTIONS

1. Preheat oven to 400 degrees.

2. If using a whole squash, pierce with a fork and microwave on high for about 5–7 minutes in order to peel and cube easier.

3. Drizzle butternut squash with oil, and roast for 30 minutes.

4. While squash is roasting, cook lasagna noodles* according to package directions. Keep them al dente.

5. While noodles* are cooking, sauté spinach in garlic and olive oil in a pan over low/medium heat.

6. In a separate bowl, combine tomato sauce with seasonings.

7. Coat a baking dish with ¼ of the tomato sauce/seasoning, and layer 3 cooked lasagna noodles* on top.

8. Put another ¼ of tomato sauce, ½ of the butternut squash, ⅓ cup ricotta* and ½ of the sautéed spinach over the noodles.

9. Continue layering ingredients in order of noodles;* ¼ of the sauce; and the other ½ of the squash, ricotta,* and spinach.

10. Put a final layer of noodles* on top, cover with the rest of the tomato sauce, and sprinkle with shredded cheese.*

11. Bake in oven for 35 minutes.

COOKING TIP

The key to this meal is making sure the butternut squash is already roasted and soft when you layer it into the lasagna. It won't soften up much during the final 35 minute cooking time.

If you want to make this dish nonvegetarian, add some ground turkey and even crumbled turkey bacon on top. Yum! This is one of the most time-consuming savory meals in this cookbook. It will take over an hour in total to prepare, so plan accordingly.

*See the appendix for allergy-friendly alternatives.

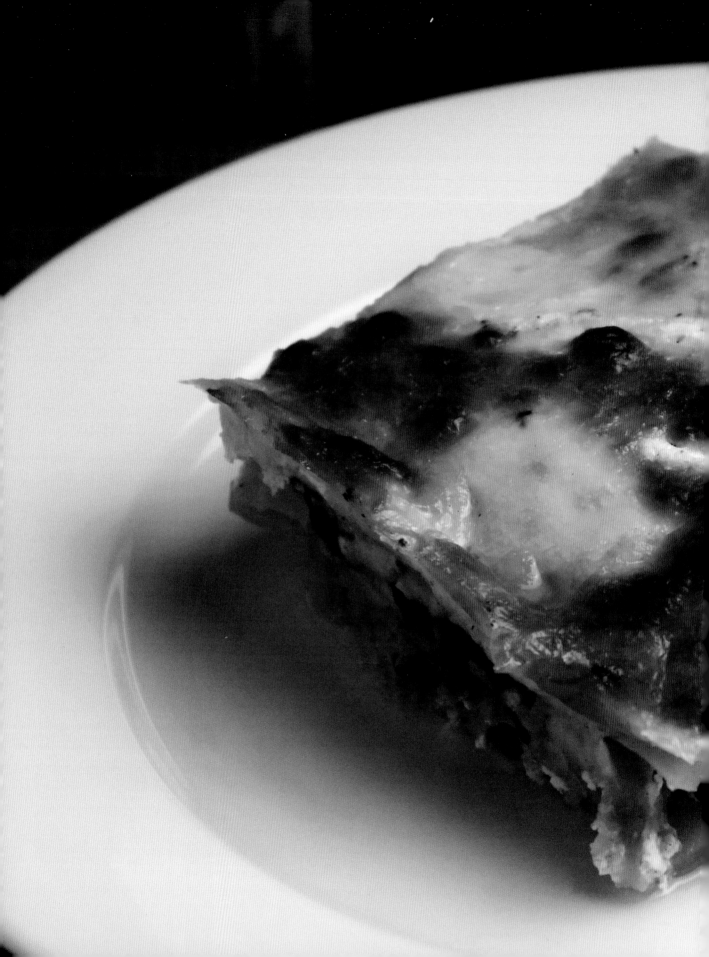

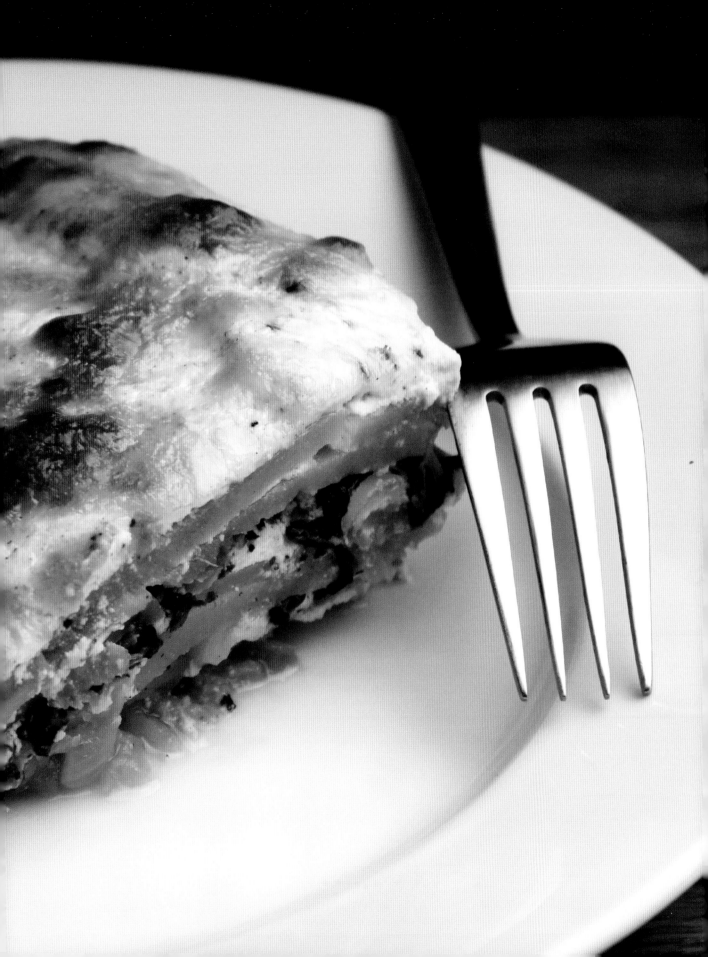

Chickpea Quinoa Veggie Bowl

Prep Time: 15 minutes
Cook Time: 25 minutes

INGREDIENTS

1 cup quinoa (uncooked)

3 T oil (split for roasting kale, broccoli, and carrots)

6 cups kale, ripped apart into small pieces

2 heads of broccoli (use just the florets)

5 large carrots, cut into small sticks

1 15-oz can of chickpeas, rinsed

DRESSING

⅓ cup olive oil

2 garlic cloves, minced

Fresh lemon juice (1/2 lemon)

Zest of one lemon

Salt, to taste

DIRECTIONS

1. Preheat oven to 400 degrees.

2. Cook quinoa according to package directions.

3. Put kale, broccoli, and carrots on separate lined baking sheets, and toss with oil and salt.

4. Roast broccoli and carrots for 20 minutes.

5. Roast kale for about 12 minutes, depending on how crisp you like it and whether other items are in the oven. If the kale is in the oven with the broccoli and carrots, you may want to roast for the whole 20 minutes as well. All ovens are slightly different. Keep an eye on the oven when roasting kale.

6. Drain and rinse chickpeas.

7. To serve, place each component of the dish (quinoa, chickpeas, carrots, broccoli, and kale) into a bowl, side by side.

8. Mix all dressing ingredients together, and drizzle on top of quinoa and vegetables.

COOKING TIP

Change up the vegetables and beans that you add to this bowl. We have tried this with kidney beans, as well as black beans. Also, roasted green beans are a great addition.

NUTRITION NOTE

This is a great meal for people who are looking for more of a plant-based eating approach. It is a favorite in our home because of the variety of foods that we combine to make this dish. There is something for everyone.

Pasta Primavera

Prep Time: 15 minutes
Cook Time: 10 minutes

INGREDIENTS

¾ lb penne pasta*

1 T oil

2 cups broccoli (fresh or frozen)

2 medium zucchinis, cut into bite-sized pieces

¼ cup water

2 cups frozen peas

3 garlic cloves, minced

Salt and pepper, to taste

1½ cups cherry tomatoes, halved lengthwise

1 T butter or butter alternative*

¼ cup grated cheese*

DIRECTIONS

1. Cook penne* according to package directions.

2. When pasta* is cooking, heat oil over low/medium heat, and sauté broccoli for 3 minutes.

3. Add zucchini to pan, and sauté for 2 more minutes.

4. Add water.

5. Add peas.

6. Add garlic, salt, and pepper, and sauté for an additional 2 minutes.

7. Stir in tomatoes and butter.*

8. When butter melts, add pasta,* and gently coat with sauce and vegetables.

9. Stir in ¼ cup grated cheese*

NUTRITION NOTE

This recipe brings in four different types of veggies (well, tomatoes are actually a fruit) and all their different nutrients, including B6; riboflavin; folate; vitamins C, K, and A; and minerals, like potassium and manganese. It's also packed with fiber. Add any other vegetables that your children may enjoy.

*See the appendix for allergy-friendly alternatives.

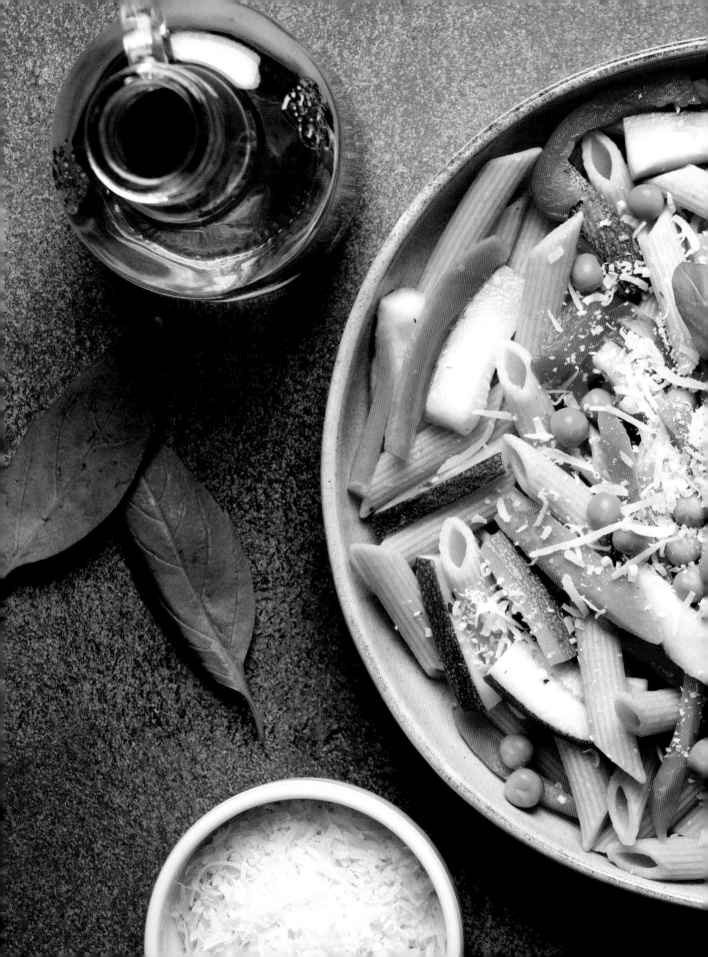

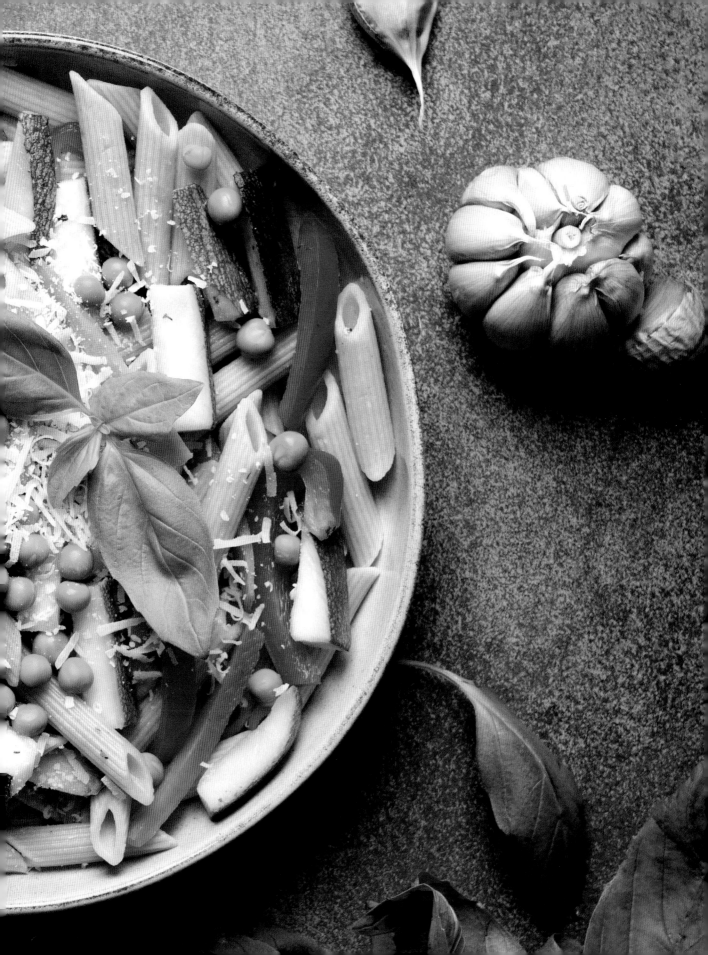

Hidden Veggie Mac and Cheese

Prep Time: 15 minutes
Cook Time: 15 minutes

INGREDIENTS

2 cups carrots, roughly chopped (about 4 carrots)

2 cups butternut squash, cubed (about half a medium squash)

1 lb elbow macaroni*

½ cup reserved vegetable water

1 cup shredded cheese*

Salt and pepper, to taste

DIRECTIONS

1. Boil carrots and squash until soft. Reserve ½ cup of vegetable water.

2. Make pasta* according to package directions.

3. Remove veggies from pot with a slotted spoon, and blend in a food processor with 1–2 T of vegetable water, until smooth. Add more water as needed.

4. When drained pasta* is still hot, pour vegetable sauce over, and stir in shredded cheese* until melted.

5. Salt and pepper, to taste. Serve immediately.

COOKING TIP

If you have leftover butternut squash, toss in oil, sprinkle with salt, and roast at 400 degrees for 20–30 minutes.

If you want even more sauce, add in more veggies. You likely won't need to add more cheese though. The vegetables are what gives the sauce its smooth consistency and volume. The cheese is there for flavor, mostly.

*See the appendix for allergy-friendly alternatives.

Stuffed Peppers

Prep Time: 5 minutes
Cook Time: 55 minutes

INGREDIENTS

1 cup quinoa (uncooked)

About 6 bell peppers

1 15-oz can of tomato sauce

½ 15-oz can of fire-roasted diced tomatoes

1 15-oz can of kidney beans

2 tsp oregano

2 tsp garlic powder

2 tsp onion powder

½ cup shredded cheese*

DIRECTIONS

1. Preheat oven to 350 degrees.

2. Cook quinoa according to package directions.

3. While quinoa is cooking, prep the peppers. Wash, cut out stems, and clean out the seeds.

4. In a large skillet on low heat, add tomato sauce, diced tomatoes, beans, and seasonings (oregano, garlic powder, and onion powder). Mix until combined.

5. Add cooked quinoa. Combine.

6. Place peppers in a baking dish or muffin tin. Balance them so they will stay upright.

7. Spoon quinoa mixture into each pepper.

8. Sprinkle shredded cheese* on the top of each pepper.

9. Bake for 40 minutes.

NUTRITION NOTE

Add a grain other than quinoa to give peppers a different taste, texture, and nutrient composition. We have used brown rice, farro, and couscous. If you are gluten-free, stick to rice, quinoa, or other gluten-free grains.

If you want a lower-carbohydrate option that is nonvegetarian, skip the grain all together, and add ground turkey.

*See the appendix for allergy-friendly alternatives.

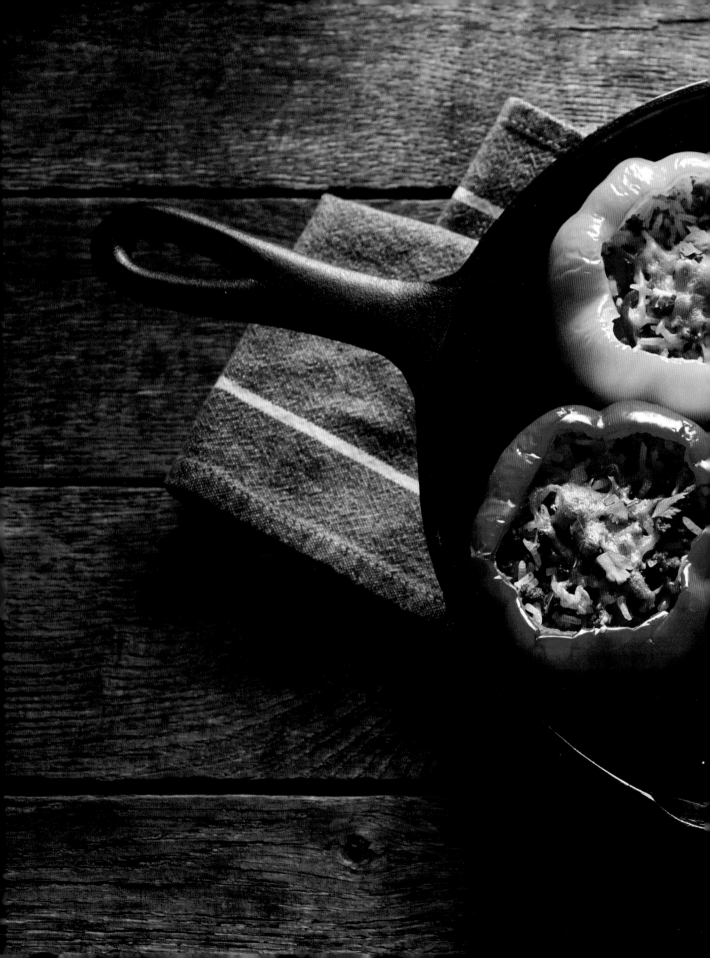

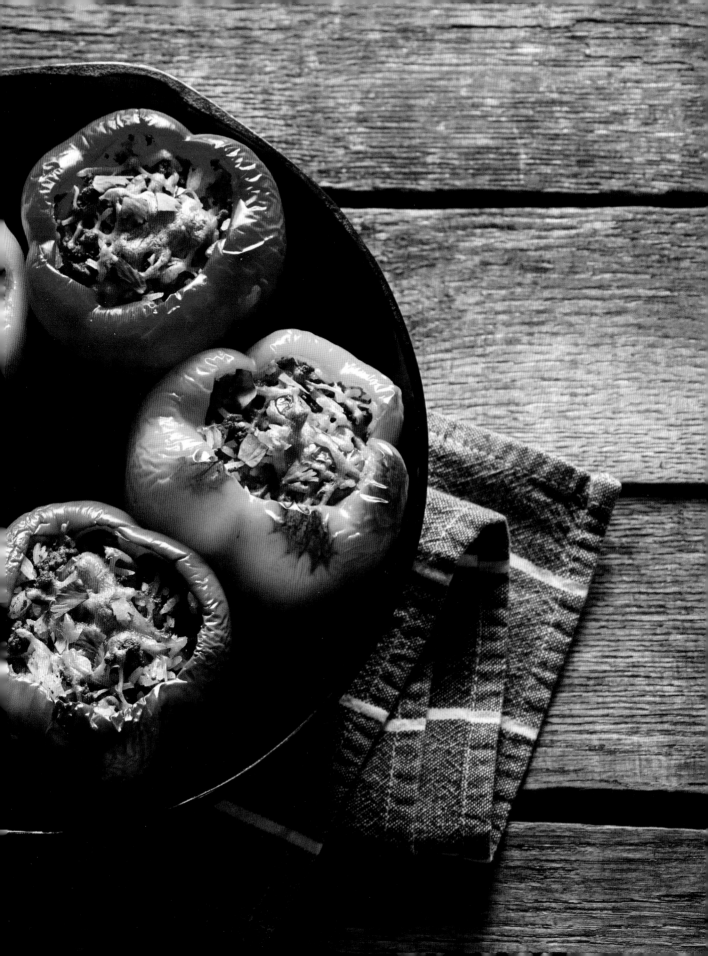

Veggie Burgers

Makes 6 burgers.
Prep Time: 10 minutes
Cook Time: 20 minutes

INGREDIENTS

2 T oil (split)

½ yellow onion, diced

1 cup portobello mushrooms, chopped

3 cups baby spinach

1 cup cooked quinoa

1 cup black beans

⅓ cup italian seasoned breadcrumbs*

2 tsp garlic powder

¼ tsp cumin

⅛ tsp smoked paprika (go up to ¼ tsp if your family likes this spice)

⅛ tsp turmeric (go up to ¼ tsp if your family likes this spice)

Salt and pepper, to taste

DIRECTIONS

1. On low/medium heat, sauté onion and mushrooms with 1 T of oil for 3–5 minutes. Add baby spinach, and cook until wilted.

2. Blend cooked veggies with all other ingredients (except the other 1 T of oil) in a food processor. If you like texture in your veggie burgers, use the pulse setting.

3. Heat 1 T oil in a pan on low/medium heat.

4. Form mixture into patty, and cook 4 minutes on each side until browned.

COOKING TIP

Be gentle when flipping patties, or they may fall apart. If you are having trouble keeping them together, opt for a slider-sized patty instead of a full-sized.

We tend to use less spice in this recipe so that our children are more likely to eat it. It all depends on your family's tastes. If your children like spice, go up to the ¼ tsp suggestion. The ⅛ tsp is very mild.

NUTRITION NOTE

This burger is delicious and very healthy. You are getting plant-based protein sources from the quinoa and beans. A great addition would be sliced avocado on top to add a healthy fat source.

*See the appendix for allergy-friendly alternatives.

Vegetarian Tacos

Prep Time: 15 minutes
Cook Time: 15 minutes

INGREDIENTS

2 T oil

½ yellow onion, diced

1 red bell pepper, diced

2 large garlic cloves, minced

1 15-oz can of kidney or cannellini beans

½ tsp cumin

1½ tsp oregano

1 cup tomato sauce

Taco shells*

Toppings: shredded cheese,* sliced avocado, diced tomatoes, red onion, and lettuce

DIRECTIONS

1. Heat oil in large pan over low/medium heat. Add diced onions and peppers. Sauté for about 3–5 minutes.

2. Add garlic. Sauté for an additional minute or until fragrant.

3. Add beans, cumin, and oregano. Combine.

4. Add tomato sauce, and turn heat down to low.

5. Simmer for an additional 5 minutes.

6. Place mixture into a gluten-free hard or soft taco shell,* and top with dairy-free shredded cheese* and other desired toppings.

NUTRITION NOTE

We sometimes make this a nonvegetarian dish and substitute the can of kidney beans with ground turkey. Also, try baking your taco shells by using a soft tortilla instead of buying premade fried shells. See recipe below. You can even ditch the shell altogether, and wrap everything in a large lettuce leaf.

*See the appendix for allergy-friendly alternatives.

Baked Taco Shells

Cook Time: 7–9 minutes

INGREDIENTS

Soft tortilla*

DIRECTIONS

1. Preheat oven to 375 degrees.

2. Place tortillas* on taco-shell maker, or drape each shell over two bars of your oven rack.

3. Bake 7–9 minutes, depending on how crunchy you want them.

*See the appendix for allergy-friendly alternatives.

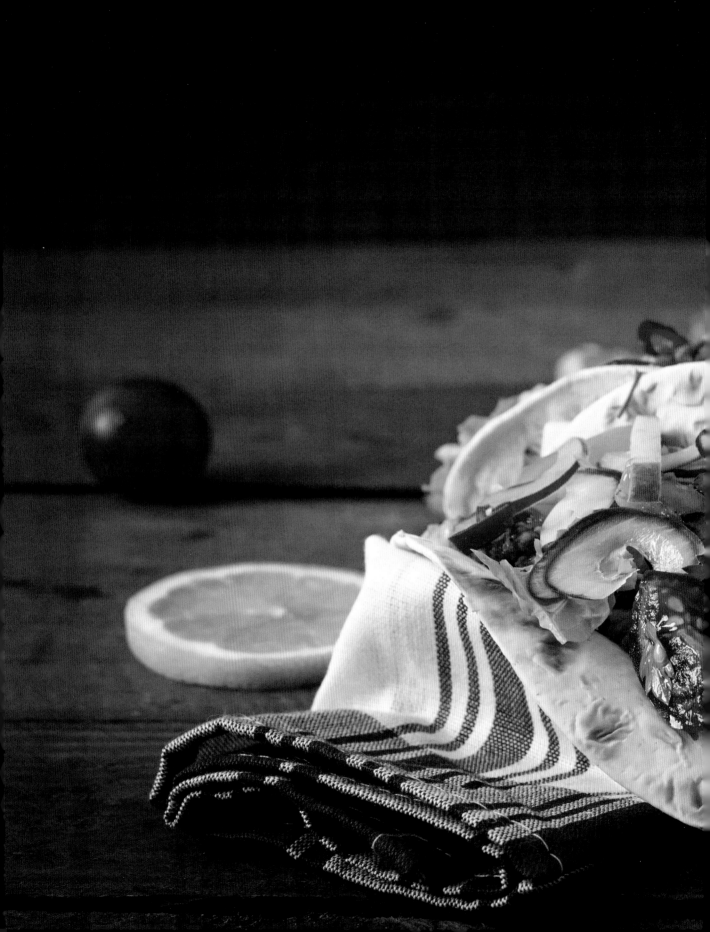

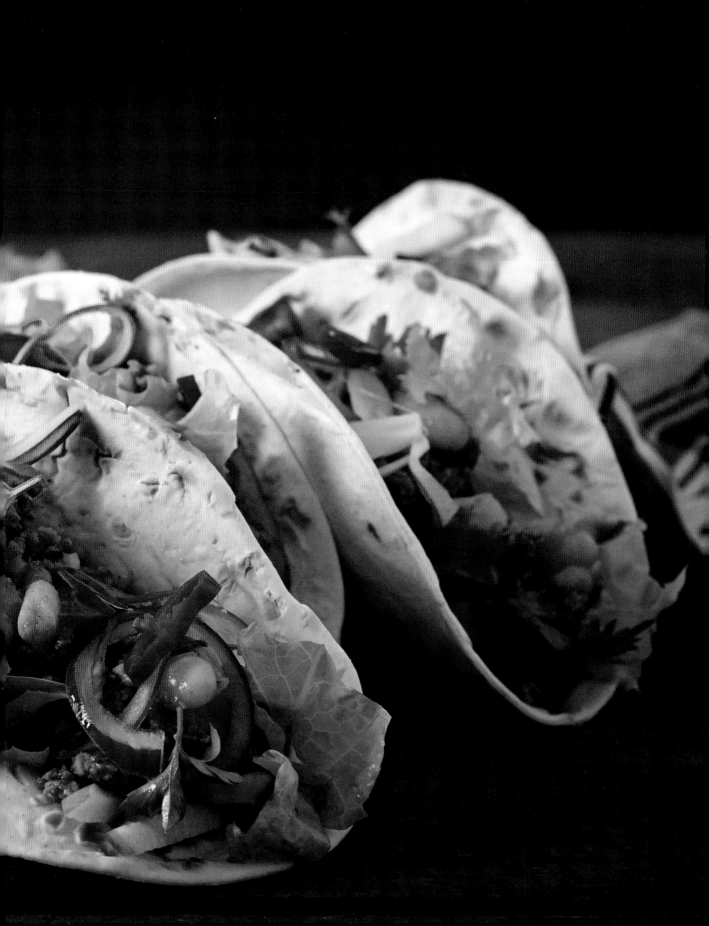

Sides and Sauces

Rather than buying premade sauces and dressings, try to make them at home. They will taste fresh and will contain no additives, fillers, excess salt, sugar, or unhealthy fat. They take a little added time but are well worth the effort.

Growing up, we always ate bottled dressing and jarred sauces, but as an allergy mom, it was easier for me to create my own sauces and dressings. I didn't want to call manufacturers or search in a grocery store for an item that wasn't even that good, especially when I could make a healthier version at home.

Butternut squash is a healthy and versatile ingredient, and several of my recipes include it. Initially, I was trying to make a butternut squash soup, but it ended up a sauce instead. In the cooking tips, I also give the directions to create a soup out of it, but our family enjoys it as a sauce even more. We randomly came upon the grape tomato sauce as well. If you start to experiment in the kitchen, you will see how often this happens. I had lots of grape tomatoes from our garden, so I decided to try using them. I ended up with another delicious sauce recipe.

My husband created the salad dressing recipe. He never measured anything out and just added the dressing directly on top of the salad at dinner, so I had to watch him closely to see how much of each ingredient he added for a single serving, and then experimented. This dressing is far superior to any store-bought dressing. It is fresh, light, healthy, and delicious.

I also created an array of veggie-based side dishes, for those who are tired of steamed broccoli as their healthy side dish. Sweet potato fries are huge in our house. They are easy to make and a much healthier version than the traditional french fry. You can use other root vegetables, such as parsnips, turnips, and white or red potatoes too.

The holidays can be difficult for families living with food allergies because we gather with family and friends who may not think of food allergies when creating the menu. When we go to others' homes for the holidays, we ask what will be served and create a safe version for our children if the host is unable to do so. This is how the herb stuffing came about. I always loved stuffing on Thanksgiving and, unfortunately, the traditional ingredients didn't work for our daughter, so I created a healthy and safe version for her that the whole family and extended family now enjoy. That's the beauty of these recipes. You may be introducing a healthier version to others who don't even have food allergies.

Butternut Squash Sauce

Prep Time: 5 minutes (if using precut squash)
Cook Time: 15 minutes

INGREDIENTS

1 small butternut squash

2 garlic cloves, peeled and whole

1 T oil

1 small yellow onion, diced

¾ cup water, reserved from boiling squash

1 tsp dried rosemary

Salt and pepper, to taste

¼ cup grated cheese* (optional)

DIRECTIONS

1. Peel squash and cut into cubes. Poke holes, and microwave on high 4 minutes in order to soften prior to cutting, or use precut squash.

2. Boil squash and whole garlic cloves until soft. Boiling garlic is key or the flavor will be too overpowering.

3. Heat 1 T oil in pan and add onion. Sauté until fragrant and a bit browned.

4. Put squash, garlic, and reserved water in a food processor, and blend until smooth. You may want to start with ½ cup water and add more, if needed, to reach your desired consistency.

5. Add sautéed onion and rosemary to food processor, and blend until smooth.

6. Salt and pepper, to taste.

7. Optional: Sprinkle with grated cheese* when serving.

COOKING TIP

If you want to make this into a soup, thin out the sauce with ½ cup chicken or vegetable broth. Add ⅛ tsp of cinnamon for a warm fall flavor. Do not add too much cinnamon, or it will overpower the other flavors. Whether as a sauce or a soup, this is a great recipe to freeze for future use.

NUTRITION NOTE

Butternut squash will supply you with a good amount of vitamins A and C, manganese, potassium, and magnesium. Use as an alternative to tomato sauce.

*See the appendix for allergy-friendly alternatives.

Grape Tomato Sauce

Prep Time: 10 minutes
Cook Time: 10 minutes

INGREDIENTS

1 T oil

3 garlic cloves, minced

1 pint of grape tomatoes, cut in half lengthwise

1 15-oz can of pure tomato sauce

2 tsp of onion powder

2 tsp of oregano

1 tsp of dried basil

1 T of tomato paste

DIRECTIONS

1. Heat oil in a large pan, and add garlic. Over low heat, sauté for 2 minutes or until fragrant.

2. Add tomatoes and tomato sauce. Cook for 1–2 minutes.

3. Add onion powder, oregano, basil, and tomato paste into pan.

4. Simmer for 5 minutes.

NUTRITION NOTE

Cooking tomatoes boosts its cancer-fighting ability by increasing the levels of beneficial phytochemicals. The heat from cooking makes the lycopene found in tomatoes more usable to the body as compared to raw tomatoes. It's important to remember that cooking tomatoes also destroys other nutrients such as beta-carotene and vitamin C. Bottom line is whether raw or cooked, tomatoes are a healthy addition to your diet.

Salad Dressing

Makes 1 serving.
Prep Time: 2 minutes

INGREDIENTS

1 T extra virgin olive oil

4 tsp white balsamic vinegar

⅛ tsp oregano

⅛ tsp garlic powder

⅛ tsp onion powder

Salt and pepper, to taste

DIRECTIONS

1. Mix oil, vinegar, and spices together in a small tasting bowl.

2. Pour over salad. Toss the salad.

3. Add salt and pepper, as desired.

COOKING TIP

By single serving, I mean this recipe is just enough if you are having a large salad as your meal. Double the recipe if you are making a side-dish salad for the entire family. When you have enough flavor through the seasonings, you don't need tons of oil.

NUTRITION NOTE

Bottled dressings contain a lot of additives, such as sugar and salt. If you can spare a couple of minutes, opt to make your own. You won't regret it.

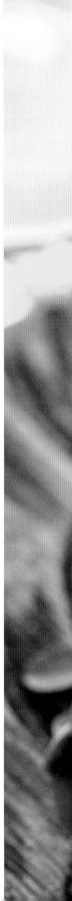

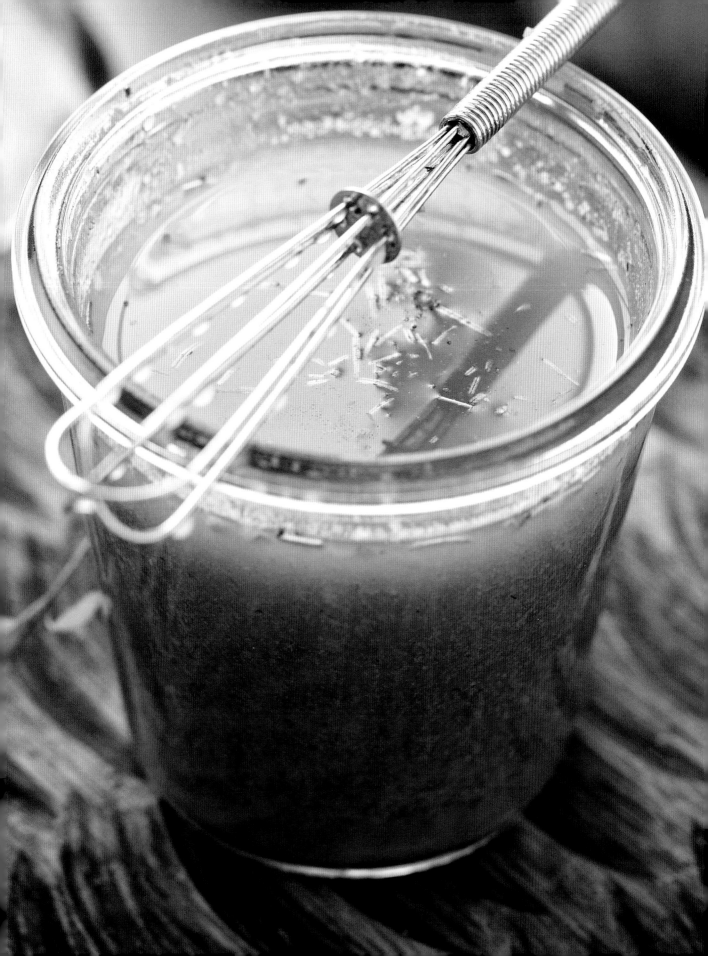

Herb Stuffing

Prep Time: 10 minutes
Cook Time: 40 minutes

INGREDIENTS

2 T of butter*

1 small to medium yellow onion, diced

5 celery stalks, diced

⅔ loaf of bread, cut into cubes*

2 tsp fresh or dried sage
  (or other herbs that you like)

Salt and pepper, to taste

2 cups low-sodium vegetable broth

DIRECTIONS

1. Preheat oven to 350 degrees.

2. Melt butter* in skillet over low/medium heat. Add onion and celery. Sauté for about 7 minutes, stirring occasionally.

3. In a large bowl, combine veggie/butter mixture, cubed bread,* sage, salt, and pepper. Toss to combine.

4. Add 2 cups of broth, and mix gently.

5. Put into casserole dish.

6. Bake for 30 minutes. This stuffing will be crispy on the top and moist underneath.

COOKING TIP

We use Alvarado's Bakery sprouted barley bread in this recipe, which is made in a nut-free facility but is not gluten free. See the appendix for gluten-free bread options.

NUTRITION NOTE

Sage is high in vitamin K and also contains minerals such as magnesium, zinc, and copper. It has a strong flavor, and, therefore, we usually use it in small amounts. Other herbs we have used in this recipe are thyme and rosemary. All of these are delicious.

*See the appendix for allergy-friendly alternatives.

Three Bean Salad

Serves 8–10
Prep Time: 15 minutes

INGREDIENTS

1 15-oz can of kidney beans

1 15-oz can of chickpeas

1 15-oz can of cannellini beans

½ red onion, diced

3 celery stalks, diced

1 red pepper, diced

1 cucumber, diced

DRESSING

¼ cup of white balsamic vinegar

2 T of olive oil

Lemon zest from 1 lemon

1 tsp garlic powder

2 tsp oregano

Salt and pepper, to taste

DIRECTIONS

1. Put all salad ingredients in a large bowl.

2. Mix all dressing ingredients and pour over salad.

3. Chill in refrigerator before serving.

COOKING TIP

You can also make the dressing on the side and add it to the salad before serving. Another nice addition could be artichoke hearts and/or beets. The options are endless.

NUTRITION NOTE

For added richness and healthy fat, slice ¼ avocado on top of each serving.

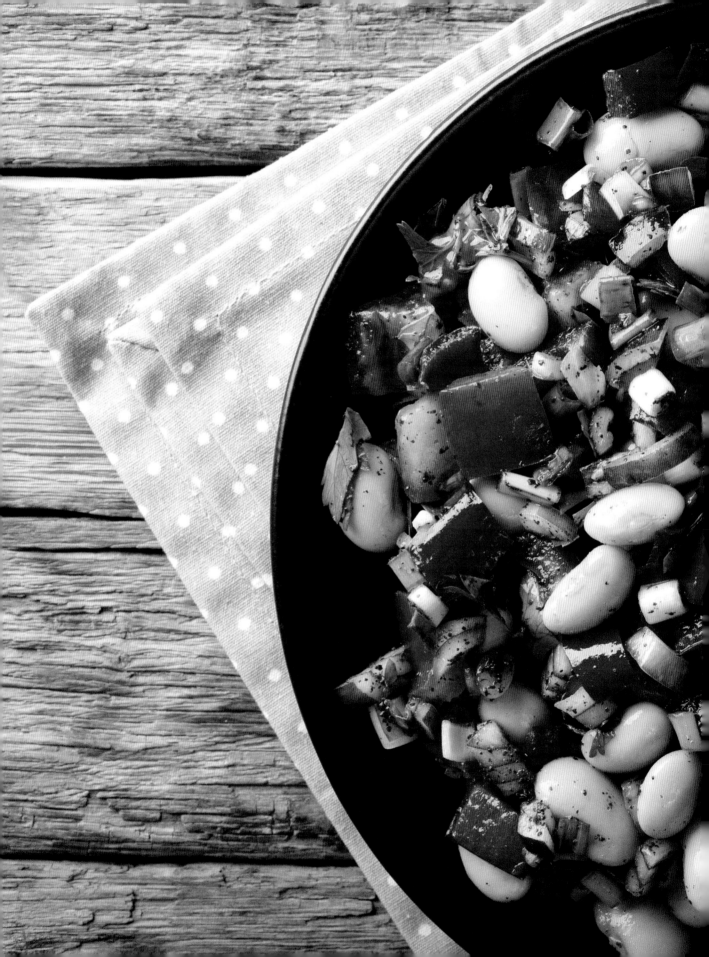

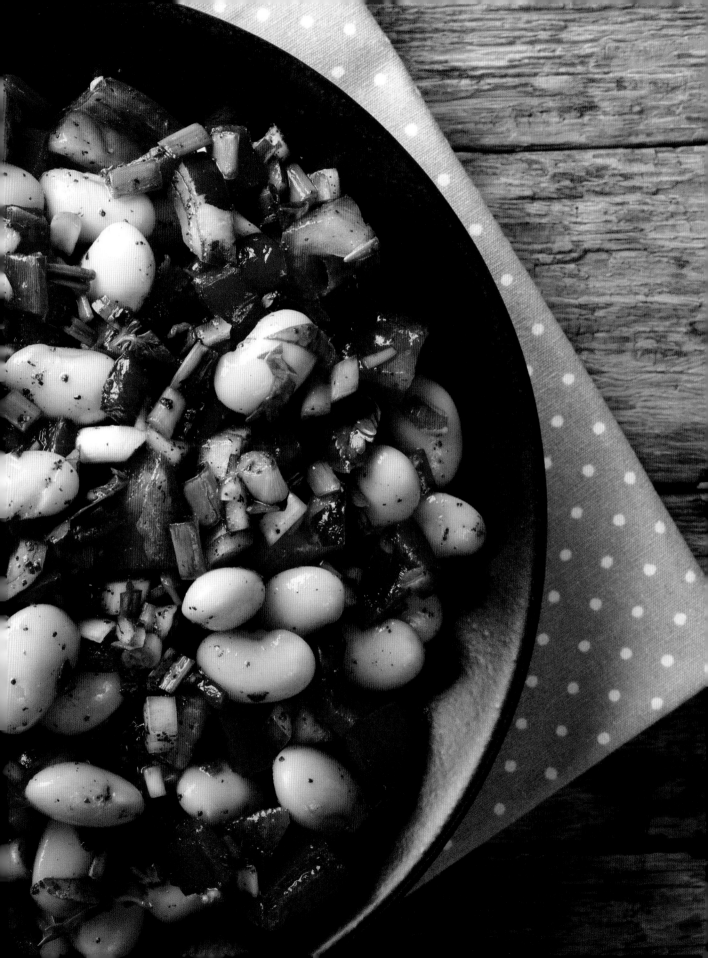

Macaroni Salad

Serves 8
Prep Time: 10 minutes
Cook Time: 20 minutes

INGREDIENTS

1 lb elbow macaroni*

1 zucchini, cut into bite-sized pieces

3 large carrots. cut into thin disks

1 red pepper, chopped into
    bite-sized pieces

3 celery stalks, chopped into
    bite-sized pieces

¼ cup olive oil

¼ cup white balsamic vinegar

1 tsp oregano

Salt and pepper, to taste

1 T lemon zest

DIRECTIONS

1. Prepare macaroni* according to package directions.

2. Put chopped veggies (zucchini, carrots, red pepper, and celery) in a large bowl, and cover with warm, cooked pasta.* Cover bowl, and let sit for at least 10 minutes. This will make the vegetables a little softer but still maintain that fresh crunch.

3. Combine olive oil, vinegar, oregano, salt, and pepper in a small bowl.

4. Pour dressing over macaroni* and veggie mixture. Combine well.

5. Add lemon zest on top.

6. Serve immediately, or keep refrigerated until ready to serve. Tastes great warm or cold.

COOKING TIP

If you do not want to make your own dressing, then any italian dressing will do. This is the perfect side dish for a summer BBQ.

This recipe calls for lemon zest because that is my preference. If you come across a recipe that calls for lemon juice, here is a useful conversion. 1 small lemon = 3 T fresh juice; 1 medium lemon = 4 T fresh juice; 1 large lemon = 5 T fresh juice. This way, if you are buying lemons for a recipe, you know how many to buy.

NUTRITION NOTE

Add beans, chicken, and/or tuna for protein.

Adding a whole bunch of varied veggies to any dish will give you the added nutrition that your body needs. In this recipe, some fun and delicious additions could be artichoke hearts or cherry tomatoes. You could even add some sliced avocado on top when serving.

*See the appendix for allergy-friendly alternatives.

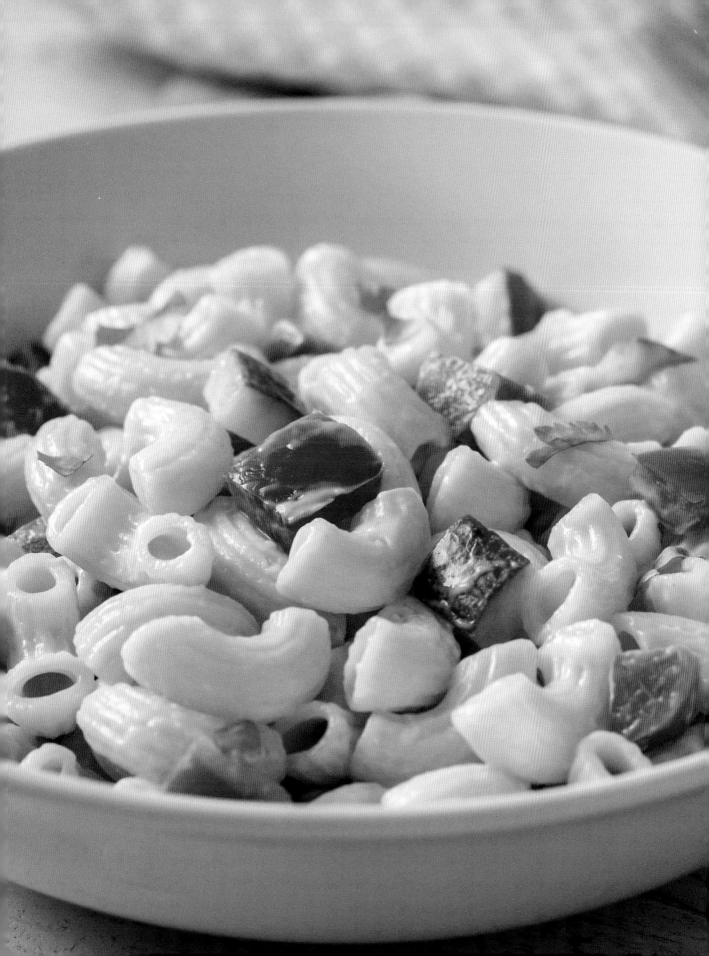

Peas and Asparagus with Thyme

Prep Time: 5 minutes
Cook Time: 20 minutes

INGREDIENTS

1 lb bunch of asparagus

2 tsp oil

8-oz bag of frozen peas

1 tsp dried thyme

Salt and pepper, to taste

DIRECTIONS

1. Preheat oven to 400 degrees.

2. Wash asparagus, and cut into 1- to 2-inch pieces. Place on foil-lined baking sheet, and combine with oil. Sprinkle with salt.

3. Bake for 20 minutes.

4. While asparagus is roasting, cook peas to package directions.

5. Combine cooked peas and asparagus in a bowl. Add thyme, salt, pepper, and mix.

COOKING TIP

I usually make this side during the fall, and thyme always makes me think of Thanksgiving, so I tend to add it. You can experiment with other herbs too, such as rosemary.

NUTRITION NOTE

Since I already spoke to the health benefits of asparagus on another nutrition note, let me tell you a little bit about peas. Peas are legumes, like lentils, chickpeas, and other beans. They are a good source of vitamins C and E, zinc, and other antioxidants that strengthen your immune system. In ½ cup of peas, you will also get 4 grams of protein. This is why you may see more vegetarian and allergy-friendly products with peas as the main source of protein.

Sweet Potato Fries

Prep Time: 10 minutes
Cook Time: 30 minutes

INGREDIENTS

2 large sweet potatoes

2–3 T oil

Garlic powder and salt, to taste.

DIRECTIONS

1. Preheat oven to 420 degrees.
2. Wash the sweet potatoes and cut into french fry–like strips.
3. Place aluminum foil on a baking sheet, and spread fries out.
4. Drizzle oil onto fries, and mix around so all strips are covered.
5. Sprinkle with garlic powder and salt.
6. Bake for 30 minutes.

COOKING TIP

To increase variety, you can use turnips, white potatoes, or parsnips instead of sweet potatoes. You can cut into cubes or disks as well. The thinner your strips, the quicker your fries will cook. Be sure to check on them after 25 minutes of baking.

NUTRITION NOTE

Rather than peeling your potatoes, keep the skin on for additional fiber and nutrition.

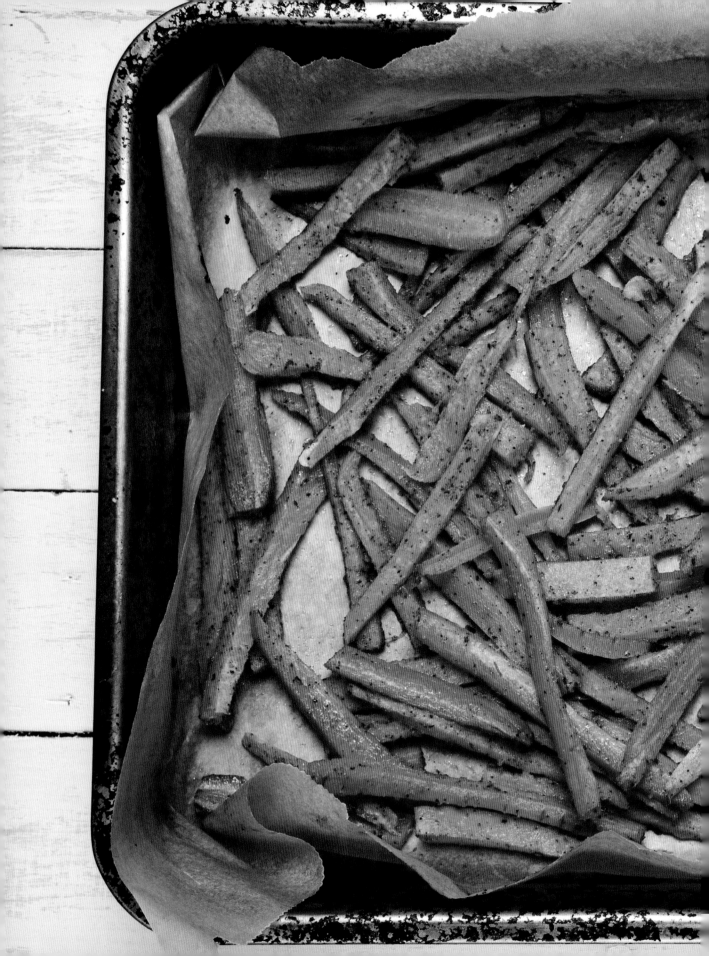

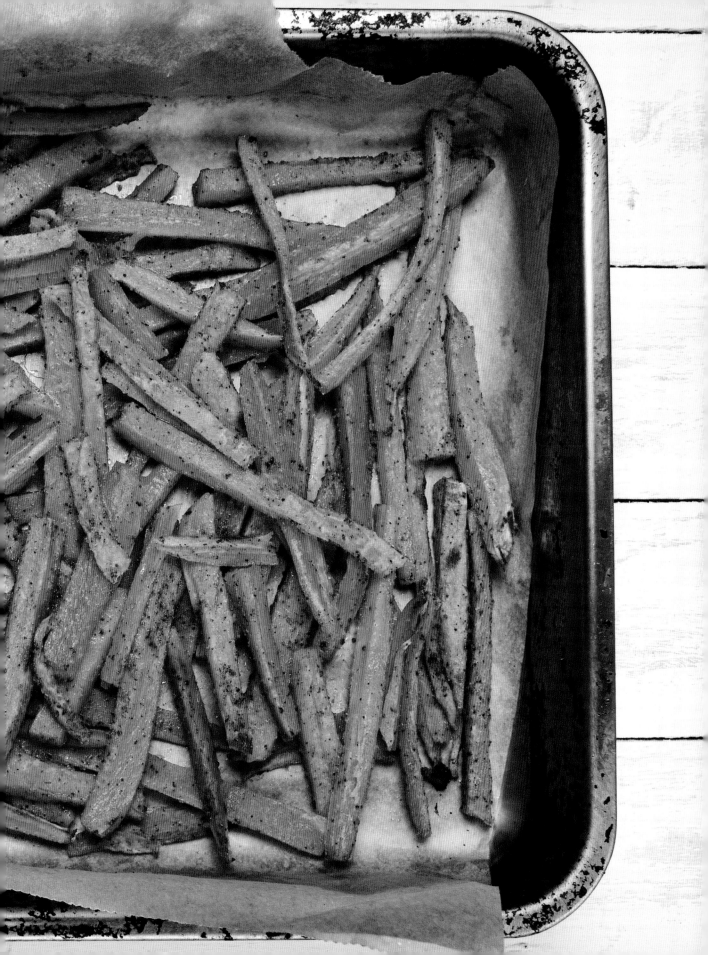

Desserts

ven though desserts are notorious for being high in sugar and unhealthy, the majority of these dessert recipes are significantly lower in sugar than traditional recipes. In many of the recipes, I have broken down the sugar content per serving, so you can understand how much your family will be getting. The goal for added sugar for a child per day is only 12 grams. A woman should aim for 24 grams or less, and a man, 36 grams of added sugar or less. I know we all read ingredient labels as food allergy parents, but we also need to be reading nutrition labels as well.

Desserts can be tricky and frustrating at times for a family living with food allergies, especially if you have an egg allergy. Eggs are in the majority of dessert recipes, as I am sure you know. After a lot of experimenting in the kitchen, we have created egg-free desserts that my children love. Even now that my daughter can have baked-in egg, she still prefers our egg-free recipes. Muffins were an easy option for us because we knew we would have leftovers and wouldn't have to constantly bake. We kept some sugar in these muffin recipes, unlike the breakfast muffins, because we were looking for a dessert-like feel.

Chocolate cake was a must with our daughter. She loves anything chocolate, so I had to figure this one out. We were using a boxed mix for a while, which was safe and delicious, but the sugar content was too high, and I knew I could create something just as good with less sugar. After a lot of trial and error, we did it. We make this chocolate cake recipe all the time, and now my daughter makes it by herself when she has a chocolate cake craving.

Ice cream was another issue for us. There are barely any ice cream brands that are made in nut-free facilities, and an ice cream shop is a no-go due to cross contamination with other allergens. Also, people don't realize that some ice creams are made with egg. We purchased an ice cream machine that was a game changer for us, but the ice cream recipe in this cookbook does not call for an ice cream machine. I wanted to create an ice cream (chocolate, of course) that you could make without an ice cream machine and without loads of sugar. The addition of sunflower seed butter to the ice cream is great due to the protein content, and the recipe has zero grams of added sugar. This was a huge win for us.

We also used to use a mix for making doughnuts but, again, the sugar content was outrageous, and we were not going to go to a doughnut shop due to cross contamination. The whole family contributed to the creation of this doughnut recipe. It involved a lot of taste testing until we figured out the best ingredients and measurements.

Apple Muffins

Makes 12 muffins.
Prep Time: 20 minutes
Cook Time: 20 minutes

INGREDIENTS

1¾ cup flour*

1 tsp baking soda

2 tsp cinnamon

¼ tsp nutmeg

¼ tsp salt

¼ cup oil

⅓ cup sugar

1 cup unsweetened applesauce

1 cup diced apples

DIRECTIONS

1. Preheat oven to 350 degrees. Line muffin tin with foil liners.

2. In a medium bowl, whisk flour,* baking soda, cinnamon, nutmeg, and salt together.

3. In a large bowl, mix oil, sugar, and applesauce together.

4. Add ⅓ dry ingredients at a time to wet ingredients until blended.

5. Add diced apples.

6. Scoop batter into muffin liners, and bake 20 minutes or until a toothpick inserted into the center of muffin comes out clean.

COOKING TIP
When using ingredients such as oil and applesauce as replacements for eggs, I like to use the muffin liners made of foil instead of paper. This way the liners don't soak up the moisture of the batter. The diced apples are a great addition for added texture and a pop of tartness.

NUTRITION NOTE
These muffins have 5.5 grams of added sugar each. This is very low for muffin recipes, which are usually loaded with sugar.

*See the appendix for allergy-friendly alternatives.

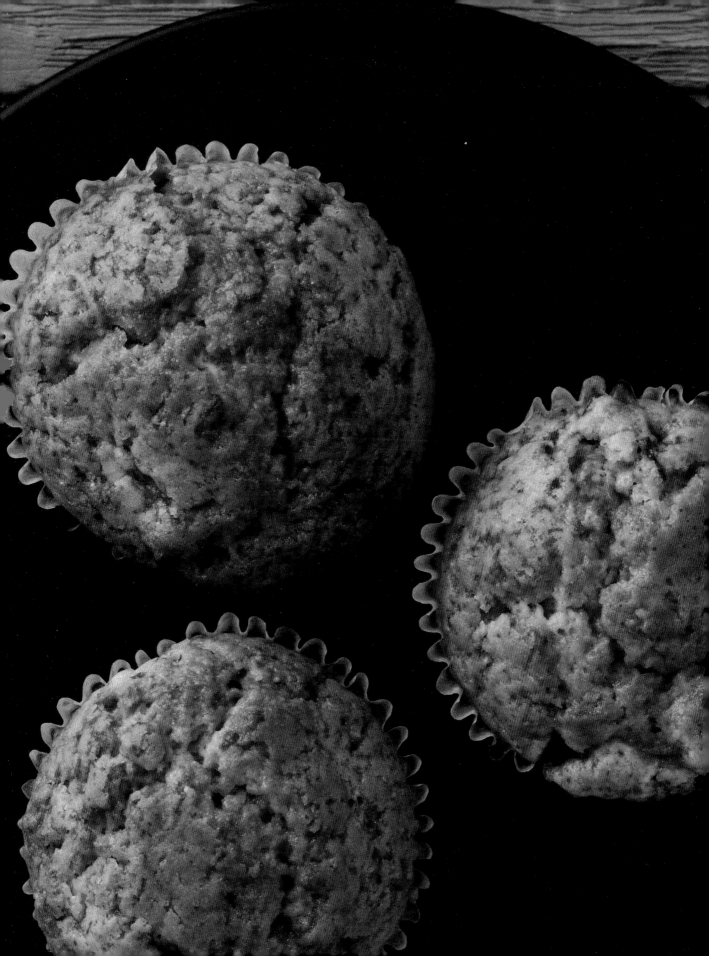

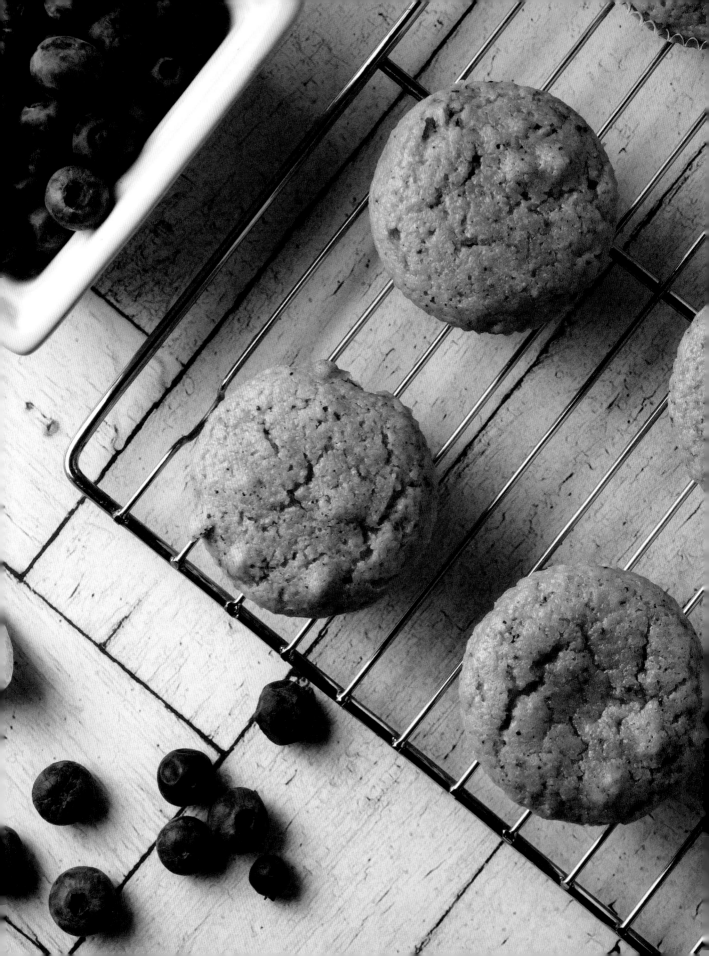

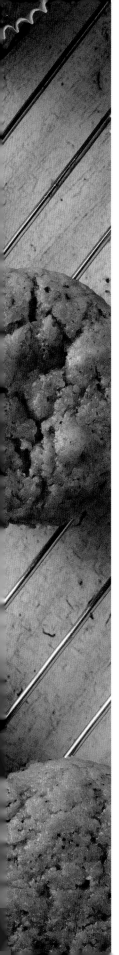

Blueberry Lemon Muffins

Makes 12 muffins.
Prep Time: 20 minutes
Cook Time: 22 minutes

INGREDIENTS

1½ cups flour*

1½ tsp baking soda

¼ tsp salt

Zest of 2 lemons

⅓ cup sugar

¾ cup milk or milk substitute*

¼ cup oil

1 T lemon juice

¾ cup fresh or frozen blueberries

DIRECTIONS

1. Preheat oven to 350 degrees, and line muffin tin with foil liners.

2. In a medium bowl, whisk together sifted flour,* baking soda, salt, and lemon zest.

3. In a large bowl, combine sugar, milk,* oil, and lemon juice. Mix until sugar is dissolved.

4. Add dry ingredients to wet ingredients; stir until just combined.

5. Fold in berries.

6. Fill muffin tins about two-thirds full.

7. Bake about 22 minutes.

8. Let cool for 5 minutes before removing from muffin tin.

NUTRITION NOTE

These are much lower in sugar than regular muffins, having a total of 5.5 grams of added sugar in each muffin.

*See the appendix for allergy-friendly alternatives.

Chocolate Cake

Prep Time: 10 minutes
Cook Time: 25 minutes

INGREDIENTS

1½ cups flour*

3 T unsweetened cocoa powder

1 tsp baking soda

⅔ cup sugar

¼ tsp salt

1 T white vinegar

¼ cup oil

1 cup water

1 tsp vanilla extract

DIRECTIONS

1. Preheat oven to 350 degrees.

2. Sift flour,* cocoa, baking soda, sugar, and salt into a large bowl. Whisk to combine.

3. Add vinegar, oil, water, and vanilla to the bowl. Mix until well combined. Pour into cake pan.

4. Bake at 350 degrees for 25 minutes. Poke a fork or toothpick in the middle to make sure cake is cooked through. If it comes out clean, it is done.

COOKING TIP

I have easily gotten away with ½ cup sugar, but people expect a chocolate cake to be sweet, so I put in a little extra for this recipe. I do try to keep sugar intake to a minimum even in desserts. It adds up quickly. If this cake is cut into sixteen slices, each slice will have 8 grams of added sugar.

NUTRITION NOTE

A child should aim for no more than 12 grams of added sugar a day. It is not a lot. Check all food labels. A teaspoon has 4 grams of sugar, so that is just three teaspoons a day for a child. An adult should stay within 6–8 teaspoons a day. If you decrease the sugar in this recipe to ½ cup, you will only have 6 grams of sugar per slice. Then, if you wanted a larger slice, you can get away with it.

*See the appendix for allergy-friendly alternatives.

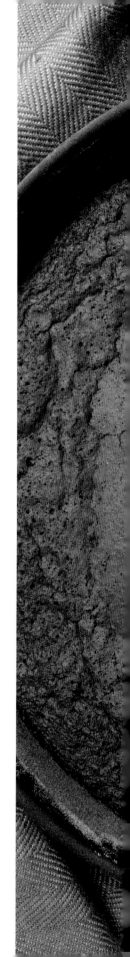

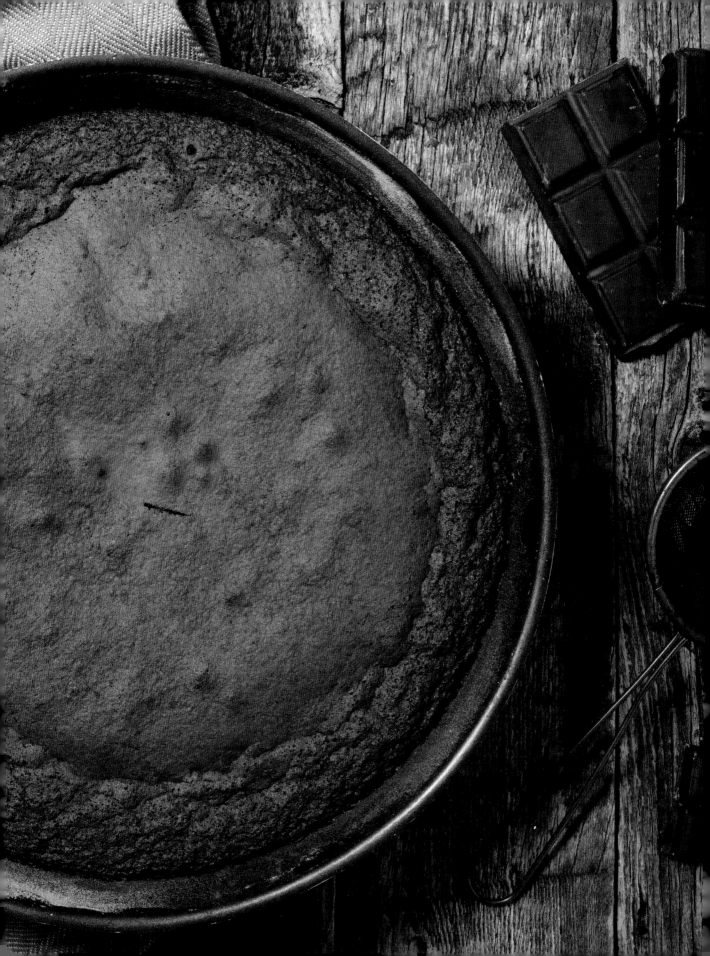

Chocolate Doughnuts

Makes about 8 doughnuts.
Prep Time: 20 minutes
Cook Time: 10 minutes

INGREDIENTS

1 cup flour*

¼ tsp baking soda

1 tsp baking powder

1½ T unsweetened cocoa powder

¼ tsp salt

¼ cup oil

⅓ cup sugar

½ cup unsweetened applesauce

¼ cup milk or milk substitute*

1 tsp vanilla

¼ cup mini chocolate chips*

DIRECTIONS

1. Preheat oven to 400 degrees.

2. In a medium bowl, sift together the flour,* baking soda, baking powder, cocoa, and salt. Whisk to combine.

3. In a large bowl, blend oil, sugar, applesauce, milk,* and vanilla. Blend with a mixer until sugar is dissolved (about 2 minutes).

4. Add half the dry ingredients to wet ingredients. Stir until just combined. Add the other half. Each time, stir just until combined. Do not overmix.

5. Mix in chocolate chips.*

6. Spoon batter into a doughnut pan until ¾ full.

7. Bake for 10 minutes.

8. Let cool for 5 minutes before removing from pan.

COOKING TIP

Why combine sugar with the wet ingredients? You want the sugar crystals to dissolve into the wet ingredients. This gives you a doughnut that is fluffy. Therefore, only in baking, sugar is considered a wet ingredient.

You can also sprinkle the mini chocolate chips on top, instead of combining them into the batter. Our family likes it both ways.

*See the appendix for allergy-friendly alternatives.

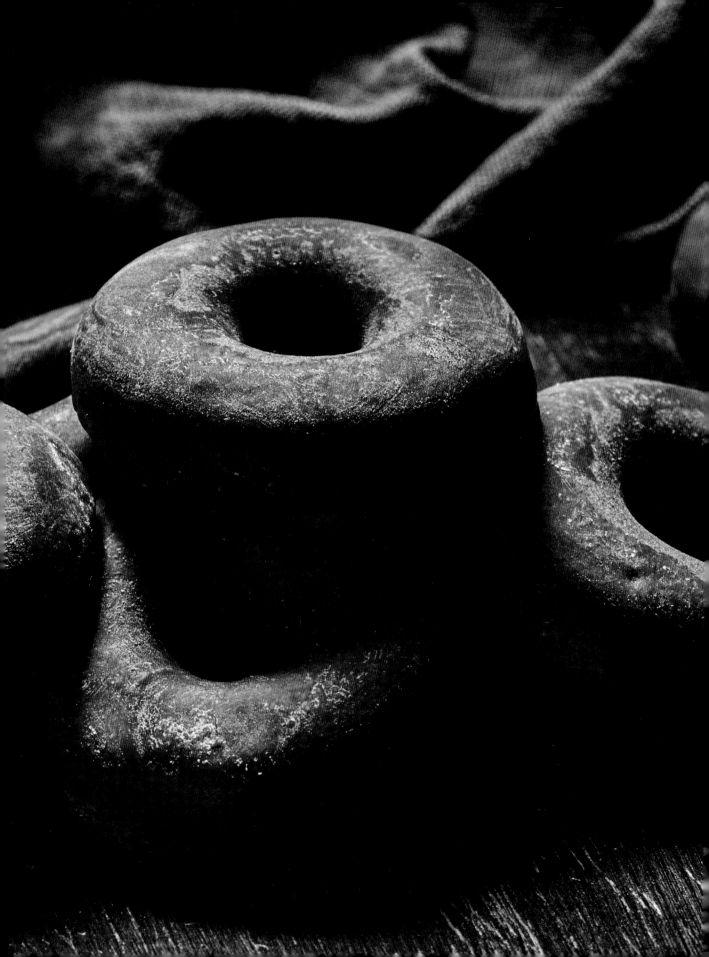

Chocolate Sunflower Butter Ice Cream

Serves 4

Prep Time: 5 minutes

Freeze Time: 2 hours

INGREDIENTS

2 very ripe bananas

1 T unsweetened sunflower butter

2 T cocoa powder

3 T milk or milk substitute*

DIRECTIONS

1. Put banana, sunflower butter, cocoa, and milk* into food processor. Blend until smooth.

2. Place into an ice cream container, and freeze for two hours.

COOKING TIP

If you leave the ice cream in the freezer for too long, it will get hard like an ice dessert, so keep an eye on the time. You can also cut up the banana into coins and freeze them prior to blending. This way you can eat the ice cream as soon as you blend it.

NUTRITION NOTE

Add fruit to top it off, and get a boost of nutrients and flavor. For added chocolatey goodness, add some mini chocolate chips.

The higher the fat content in your milk choice, the creamier the ice cream will be.

*See the appendix for allergy-friendly alternatives.

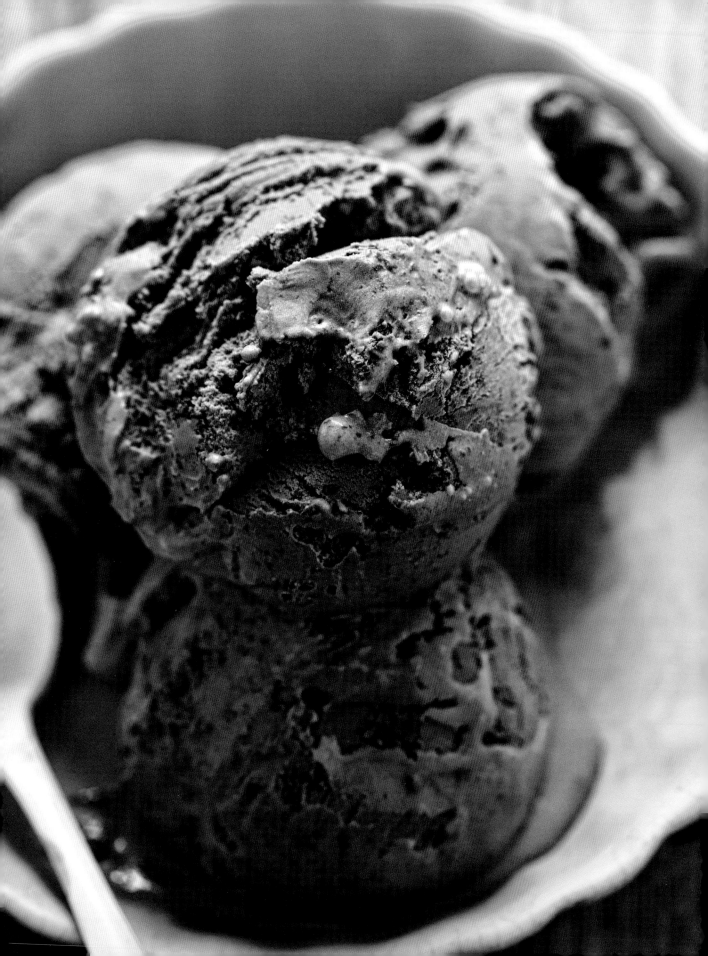

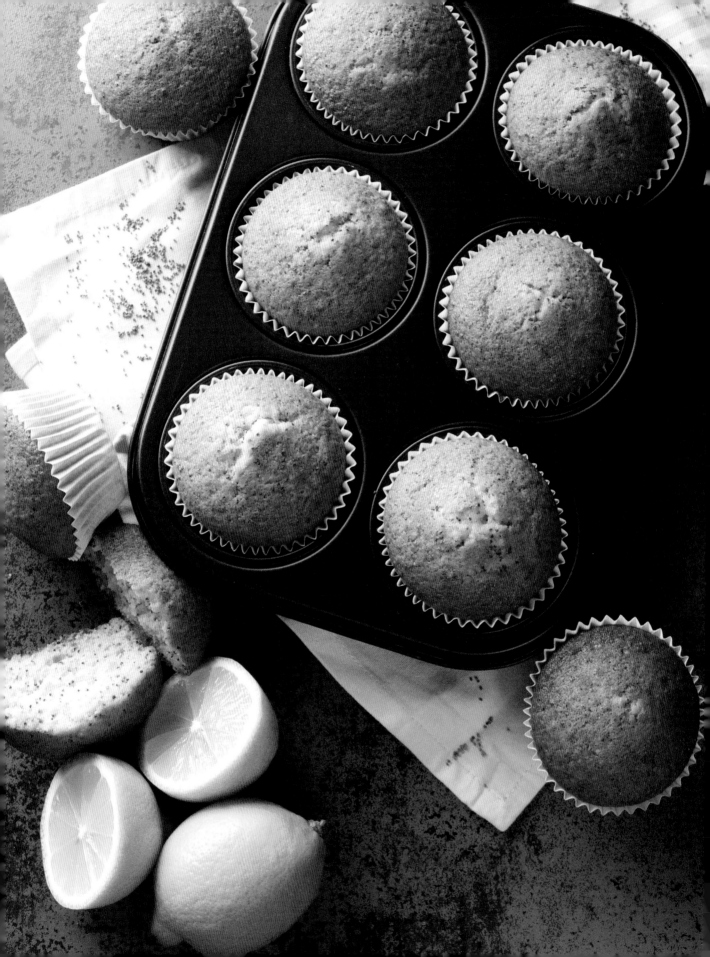

Lemon Poppy Seed Muffins

Makes 12 muffins.
Prep Time: 15 minutes
Cook Time: 25 minutes

INGREDIENTS

1 cup milk or milk substitute*

¼ cup fresh lemon juice
(approximately the juice
of one lemon)

2 cups flour*

1 T poppy seeds

2 tsp baking powder

¼ teaspoon salt

⅓ cup unsweetened applesauce

¼ cup oil

½ cup sugar

Lemon zest from 2 lemons

DIRECTIONS

1. Preheat oven to 375 degrees.

2. Line a muffin tin with liners.

3. In a medium-sized bowl, mix together milk,* and lemon juice. Set aside.

4. In another medium-sized bowl, whisk together flour,* poppy seeds, baking powder, and salt.

5. Add applesauce, oil, sugar, and lemon zest to the milk/lemon-juice mixture. Stir until sugar dissolves.

6. Pour wet ingredients into dry ingredients, and stir until just combined.

7. Scoop mixture into muffin tin. Bake 25 minutes.

8. Let cool for 5–10 minutes before eating. If muffins are too warm, the liner may not peel away as easily.

NUTRITION NOTE

My family likes this recipe with only ⅓ cup of sugar. It is very lightly sweetened this way. Others may prefer it a little sweeter because of the lemon, but give the lower sugar option a try. There are 8 grams of added sugar per muffin, as written. If you are using ⅓ cup of sugar, then there will be 5.5 grams of added sugar per muffin.

*See the appendix for allergy-friendly alternatives.

Pear & Apple Crumble

Prep Time: 20 minutes to chop the fruit
Cook Time: 40 minutes

INGREDIENTS

6 pears

6 apples

4 T butter or butter substitute*
(separated 1 T and 3 T)

2 tsp cinnamon

⅔ cup oats

1½ T brown sugar

DIRECTIONS

1. Peel pears and apples, and cut them into bite-sized pieces.

2. Add fruit to a large saucepan over low/medium heat with 1 T butter or butter substitute.*

3. Preheat oven to 350 degrees.

4. Cook fruit down on low/medium heat until fruit is soft and gooey (about 15 minutes), stirring occasionally.

5. Add cinnamon, and stir to combine.

6. Topping: In a small bowl, mix together oats and brown sugar. Pour 3 T of melted butter* over the top, and mix it all together, making sure all the oats are coated.

7. Put fruit into a 9-inch round baking dish, and sprinkle with topping.

8. Bake for 20 minutes.

COOKING TIP

We use Fuji apples and Bartlett pears for this recipe, but just about any apple or pear will do the trick.

*See the appendix for allergy-friendly alternatives.

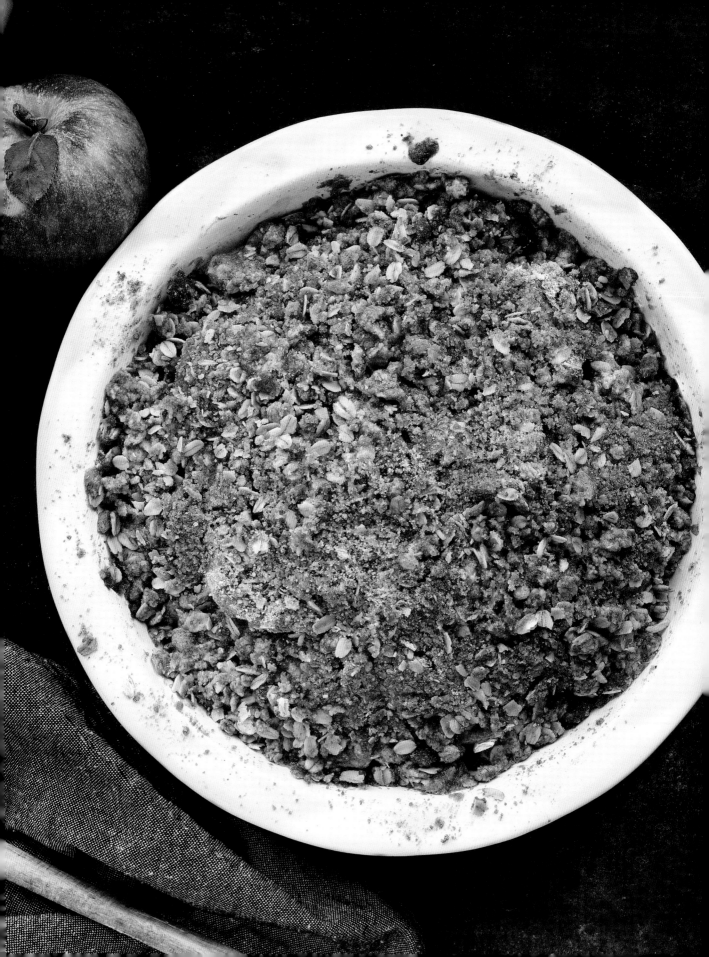

Pumpkin Cake Bars

Makes 15 servings.
Prep Time: 15 minutes
Cook Time: 30 minutes

INGREDIENTS

2 ounces cream cheese*

2 tsp baking soda

2 T white vinegar

1 cup pumpkin puree

⅓ cup sugar

1 tsp vanilla

¼ cup oil

1 cup flour*

1 tsp baking powder

1½ tsp pumpkin pie spice
(includes cinnamon, ginger,
nutmeg, and allspice)

1½ tsp cinnamon

⅛ tsp salt

DIRECTIONS

1. Preheat oven to 350 degrees. Line a baking dish (8 × 10 inch) with parchment paper. You can also prepare the baking dish with oil or butter.* For this recipe, we prefer using parchment paper for easy bar removal.

2. Melt cream cheese* in microwave on high (about 20 sec).

3. In a small bowl, stir baking soda and vinegar until combined.

4. In a large bowl, combine pumpkin puree, sugar, vanilla, cream cheese,* oil, and baking soda/vinegar mixture. Mix until combined. You can use a hand mixer to get all lumps out.

5. In a medium bowl, stir together the dry ingredients (flour,* baking powder, pumpkin pie spice, cinnamon, and salt).

6. Add dry ingredients to wet ingredients, and stir until combined. Do not over stir.

7. Pour batter into baking dish. Bake 30 minutes. Stick a toothpick or fork into center to make sure it's done.

8. Let cool at least 10 minutes before cutting into bars and serving.

NUTRITION NOTE
If you cut into 15 bars, there are 4.4 grams of added sugar per bar.

*See the appendix for allergy-friendly alternatives.

Zucchini Bread

Prep Time: 15 minutes (not including grating of zucchini)
Cook Time: 50–55 minutes

INGREDIENTS

1 tsp oil

1¾ cups flour*

1¼ tsp baking soda

1¼ tsp ground cinnamon

¼ tsp nutmeg**

¼ tsp allspice

¼ tsp salt

⅓ cup sugar

1 tsp vanilla

½ cup unsweetened applesauce

⅓ cup oil

2 cups zucchini, grated
   (2 small to medium zucchinis)

⅓ cup mini chocolate chips*

DIRECTIONS

1. Preheat oven to 350 degrees. Grease a loaf pan with oil, and set aside.

2. Whisk flour,* baking soda, cinnamon, nutmeg, allspice, and salt in a large mixing bowl.

3. In a separate mixing bowl, combine sugar, vanilla, applesauce, and oil.

4. Stir zucchini into the wet ingredients.

5. Add the wet mixture to the dry, and stir until combined. Add chocolate chips.*

6. Pour batter into loaf pan.

7. Bake for 50–55 minutes or until a toothpick you insert into the bread comes out clean.

8. Let cool at least 10 minutes. Remove from loaf pan, and enjoy.

COOKING TIP

Most zucchini and banana bread recipes call for at least 1 cup of sugar. Almost all my recipes cut the sugar significantly, and this one is not any different. It is still considered a dessert, but your sugar intake will be much lower than with any other homemade or store-bought zucchini bread. Plus, it is still delicious.

*See the appendix for allergy-friendly alternatives.

**Nutmeg is a spice that is derived from seeds, not nuts. People with a tree-nut allergy should be able to safely consume it. Of course, always check with your doctor.

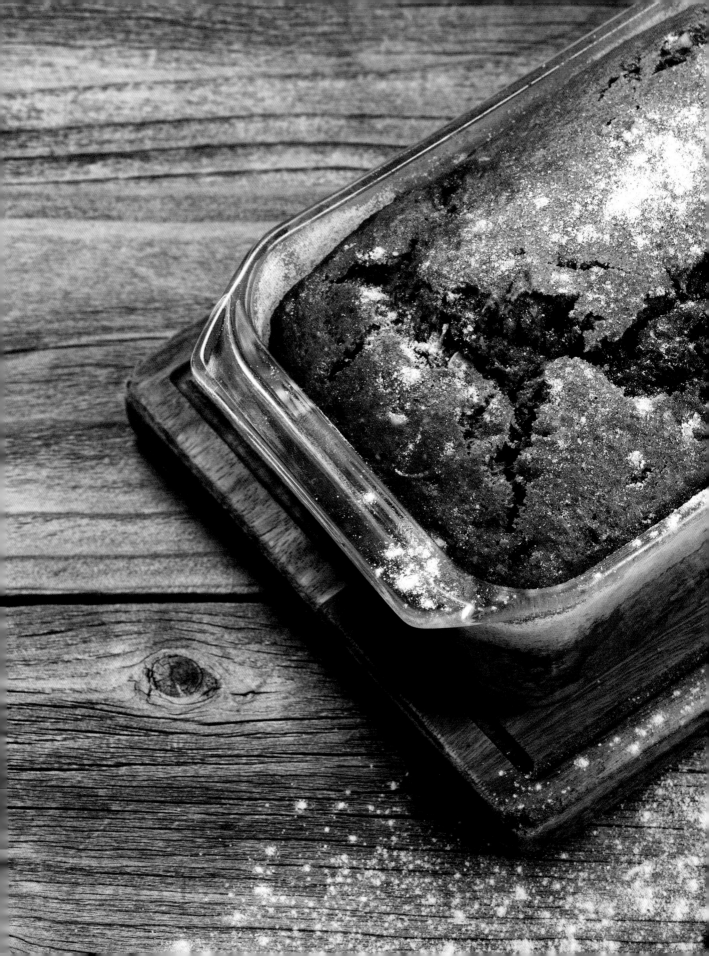

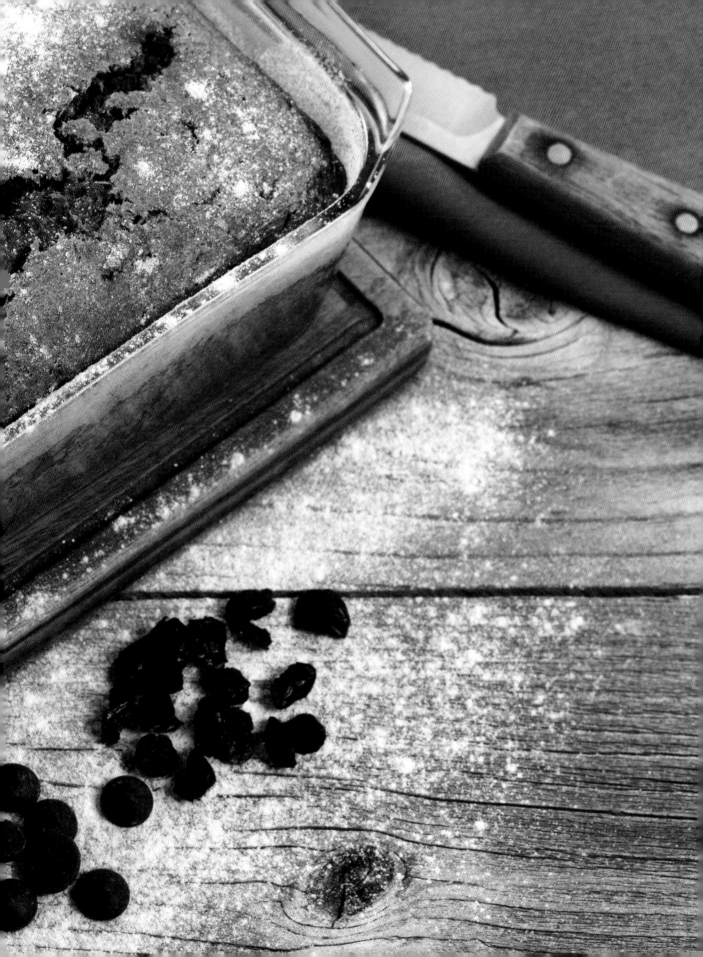

APPENDIX

Disclaimer: Brands and manufacturers change their ingredients and claims all the time. Always read the entire food label carefully every single time before using a product.

These lists are a starting point for you. Our family uses these brands and manufacturers currently, but every family has a different comfort level with shared lines and shared facilities. You'll need to contact every company—even those listed in this appendix—and ask what their practices are.

In the United States, the law does not require companies to label for shared facilities or shared lines with the top nine allergens. The only way to know if the allergen is present in the facility is if the company chooses to label with a "may contain" or "processed in the same facility as" statement. If nothing is on the food label, you must call and/or email them. My recommendation is to email so you have the company's answer in writing. If the answer is not sufficient, then you can call and speak to someone for clarification. I sometimes call twice to see if I receive the same answer. Unfortunately, I have gotten different responses from the same company, and then I do not use the product.

I have included the website associated with each product for your reference.

The first section is a list of the packaged ingredients our family uses for the recipes in this cookbook. The list is not necessarily all gluten or dairy-free, as our family does not have these two allergies, but the section that follows lists gluten- and dairy-free options.

Again, this is only a jumping-off point for you in your research for safe brands for your family. I was hesitant to add this section, since claims frequently change, but when I was first trying to navigate the allergy world, a list like this would have saved me so much time. When choosing brands, do contact each manufacturer, so you are comfortable in your decision of what to feed your family.

Brand Recommendations

APPLESAUCE

Nature's Promise 1-877-846-9949

Santa Cruz www.santacruzorganic.com. This is not a nut-free facility, but they say they will have a "may contain" statement if they feel there is a risk of cross contamination.

ARTICHOKES

Laurel Hill www.laurelhillfoods.com

Native Forest www.hivebrands.com

AVOCADO OIL

Chosen Foods www.chosenfoods.com

Pompeian www.pompeian.com

Primal Kitchen www.primalkitchen.com

BACON

Applegate www.applegate.com

BAKING POWDER

Argo www.argostarch.com

BAKING SODA

Arm & Hammer www.armandhammer.com

BEANS

Eden Organic www.edenfoods.com

Goya www.goya.com. Beans are produced in a nut-free facility, but not all Goya products are.

Nature's Promise 1-877-846-9949

BREAD

Alvarado Bakery www.alvaradostreetbakery.com

Angelic Bakehouse www.angelicbakehouse.com
See gluten-free options.

BREADCRUMBS

Gillian's www.gilliansfoodsglutenfree.com

BROTH/STOCK

College Inn www.collegeinn.com

BUTTER

Challenge www.challengedairy.com
See dairy-free options.

CANNED PUMPKIN

Libby's www.libbys.com

CHEESE

Sargento www.sargento.com
See dairy-free options.

CHOCOLATE CHIPS

Enjoy Life www.enjoylifefoods.com

COCOA POWDER

Hershey's www.thehersheycompany.com. The company will label
for possible cross contamination with any top allergens.

COW'S MILK

Nature's Promise 1-877-846-9949
See dairy-free options below.

CREAM CHEESE

Challenge www.challengedairy.com.
See dairy-free options.

DELI MEATS

Applegate www.applegate.com

FLOUR

King Arthur www.kingarthurbaking.com/allergen-program. Make sure to look
carefully at the website. Some products are gluten-free, and some are made in a
nut-free facility, while others are not. See additional gluten-free options.

FROZEN FRUIT

Wyman's www.wymans.com

GRATED CHEESE

Locatelli www.locatelli.com
See dairy-free options.

HONEY
Crystals Honey www.crystalsrawhoney.com

KETCHUP
Nature's Promise 1-877-846-9949

OATS/OATMEAL
Oats in Coats www.oatsincoats.com. Gluten-free as well.

Woodstock www.woodstock-foods.com. Not certified gluten-free. See additional gluten-free options.

OLIVE OIL
Filippo Berio www.filippoberio.com

Pompeian www.pompeian.com

PASTA
Banza www.eatbanza.com

Bionaturae www.bionaturae.jovialfoods.com

Delallo www.delallo.com. They also have gluten-free pasta, including orzo.

Ronzoni www.ronzoni.com

Tinkyada www.tinkyada.com

POPPY SEEDS
McCormick www.mccormick.com

QUINOA
Ancient Harvest www.ancientharvest.com

RICOTTA
Galbani www.galbani.com
See dairy-free options.

SPICES
McCormick www.mccormick.com

SUGAR
Domino www.dominosugar.com

SUNFLOWER SEED BUTTER
SunButter www.sunbutter.com

TOMATOES

Muir Glen www.muirglen.com
Nature's Promise 1-877-846-9949

TORTILLAS

Angelic Bakehouse www.angelicbakehouse.com
See gluten-free options.

VINEGAR

Pompeian www.pompeian.com

Gluten-Free Substitutes

Disclaimer: Brands and manufacturers change their ingredients and claims all the time. Always read the entire food label carefully every single time before using a product.

BAKING POWDER

Argo www.argostarch.com

BREAD

Gillian's Foods www.gilliansfoodsglutenfree.com
Katz www.katzglutenfree.com
Kinnikinnick www.kinnikinnick.com

BREADCRUMBS

Gerbs www.mygerbs.com
Gillian's Foods www.gilliansfoodsglutenfree.com

ENGLISH MUFFINS

Katz www.katzglutenfree.com

FLOUR

Gerbs www.mygerbs.com
Hungry Harry's www.hungryharrys.com
King Arthur www.kingarthurbaking.com/allergen-program

HAMBURGER BUNS

Gillian's Foods www.gilliansfoodsglutenfree.com
Katz www.katzglutenfree.com

OATS
Gerbs www.mygerbs.com

PASTA
Banza www.eatbanza.com
Tinkyada www.tinkyada.com

TORTILLAS
BFree www.bfreefoods.com

Dairy-Free Substitutes

Disclaimer: Brands and manufacturers change their ingredients and claims all the time. Always read the entire food label carefully every single time before using a product.

BUTTER
1 cup butter = ¾ cup vegetable or coconut oil or pureed pumpkin
1 stick of butter = 6 T unsweetened applesauce with 2 T vegetable oil
Avocado—use an equal amount
MELT butter www.meltorganic.com. This contains coconut.
For sautéing, use chicken and vegetable broths/stocks
For baking, use vegetable shortening

CREAM CHEESE
Daiya Cream Cheeze www.daiyafoods.com

GRATED PARMESAN
Follow Your Heart www.followyourheart.com

MILK
Some of these milks, such as banana, hemp, and quinoa milk, can be made at home. Manufacturers sell them as well, but several have other top allergens in their facilities.
Banana milk
Coconut milk—considered a tree nut by the FDA. If you're allergic to tree nuts, talk to your allergist before consuming
Hemp milk
Nut milk—almond and cashew are the most popular, if you don't have a nut allergy
Oat milk—www.ripplefoods.com
Pea milk—www.ripplefoods.com

Quinoa milk

Rice milk

Soy milk—if you don't have a soy allergy

RICOTTA

Use 1 oz of Daiya shreds for every ¼ cup of ricotta the recipe calls for.
www.daiyafoods.com

SLICED OR SHREDDED CHEESE

Daiya www.daiyafoods.com

Follow Your Heart www.followyourheart.com

Good Planet Foods www.goodplanetfoods.com

Egg Substitutes

Replacing eggs in a recipe can be tricky and will require some trial and error. The last few options I have found are good for leavening in a baked good. The others are a little better at binding. You do have options, so continue to experiment.

1 egg equals:

- ¼ cup applesauce, mashed avocado, or pumpkin puree
- ¼ cup vegetable oil
- ½ of a medium banana, mashed
- 2 T water, 1 T oil, and 2 tsp baking powder
- Flax egg—1 T ground flaxseeds (if no flaxseed allergy) mixed with 3 T warm water. Let stand 1 minute before using.
- 2 T arrowroot powder mixed with 3 T of water.
- 3 T aquafaba, or the liquid found in canned beans. Chickpea liquid works the best. This works as a substitute for 1 egg or 1 egg white.
- ¼ cup of carbonated water
- 1 T unflavored gelatin mixed with 1 T warm water. Pour 2 T of hot water over the mixture, and whisk vigorously. Let the gelatin "egg" sit for 2–3 minutes before adding to the recipe. This will work to substitute up to 3 eggs in a recipe.
- ¼ cup yogurt (if you don't have a dairy allergy). This is best for leavening.
- 1 tsp of baking soda mixed with 1 T of distilled vinegar. This combination works well in baked goods that are light and airy.
- Commercial egg replacement products, if using eggs primarily as a leavening agent for baked goods. Combine 1½ tsp of powder with 2–3 T of water.

Allergy-Friendly Companies

Disclaimer: Brands and manufacturers change their ingredients and claims all the time. Always read the entire food label carefully every single time before using a product.

Below is a list of allergy-friendly companies that we have used. There are many amazing companies out there that I have not tried yet. As you do your own research, you will find many more.

Enjoy Life www.enjoylifefoods.com
- Sweets and snacks that are gluten-free and free from the fourteen most common food allergens.

Free2be www.free2befoods.com
- Snacks free from the twelve most common allergens.

Gerbs www.mygerbs.com
- Selection of products free from the twelve most common food allergens.

Hilary's www.hilaryseatwell.com
- Every product is free from the top twelve most common allergens and is made from plant-based ingredients. Products include veggie burgers, whole-grain medleys, meatless sausages, and veggie bites.

Hungry Harry's www.hungryharrys.com
- Baking mixes that are free from the top fourteen food allergens and manufactured in a facility free of the top fourteen allergens.

Katz www.katzglutenfree.com
- Bakery items produced in a dedicated gluten-, dairy-, and nut-free facility. They are working to remove soy from their product line.

Kinnikinnick www.kinnikinnick.com
- Breads, bagels, cookies, buns, donuts, muffins, waffles, baking mixes, pizza, and pie crusts. Free from top eight allergens and gluten-free.

Made Good www.madegoodfoods.com
- All snacks are free from the most common allergens.

Namaste Foods www.namastefoods.com
- Baking mixes that are free from the top nine allergens.

Pascha www.paschachocolate.com
- Chocolate that is free from major food allergens.

Safe & Fair www.safeandfair.com
- Ingredients free from the top nine allergens.

Sensitive Sweets Bakery www.sensitivesweets.com
- Allergy-friendly bakery that is free of the top ten allergens and ships within the US.

Vermont Nut Free www.vermontnutfree.com
- Sweets that are produced and packaged in a dedicated nut-free facility. They do make

products in their facility that contain dairy, soy, egg, and wheat/gluten, but they will label products that were made on shared equipment.

Yum Earth www.yumearth.com
· Allergy-friendly sweets that are free of the top nine allergens and gluten-free.

Helpful Websites for the Allergy Community

AllergyEats allergyeats.com
· A peer-reviewed directory of restaurants that was launched in 2010 in order to find allergy-friendly restaurants across the United States.

American Academy of Allergy Asthma & Immunology AAAAI.org
· The leading membership organization of more than seven thousand allergists/immunologists and patients' trusted resources for allergies, asthma, and immune deficiency disorders.

American College of Allergy, Asthma, & Immunology ACAAI.org
· A professional medical association of more than six thousand allergists/immunologists and allied health professionals. Members live and practice throughout the United States and internationally.

Asthma and Allergy Foundation of America AAFA.org
· A not-for-profit organization founded in 1953, AAFA is the leading patient organization for people with asthma and allergies and the oldest asthma and allergy patient group in the world.

Food Allergy & Anaphylaxis Connection Team (FAACT) foodallergyawareness.org
· FAACT's mission is to educate, advocate, and raise awareness for all individuals and families affected by food allergies and life-threatening anaphylaxis.

Food Allergy Research & Education (FARE) foodallergy.org
· FARE's mission is to improve the quality of life and health of those living with food allergy and to provide hope for the development of new treatments. FARE has turned over $100 million in donor gifts into groundbreaking research and has provided a voice for the community.

Kids with Food Allergies (KFA) kidswithfoodallergies.org
· KFA is a division of the Asthma and Allergy Foundation of America (AAFA). KFA is dedicated to saving lives and reducing the burden of food allergies through support, advocacy, education, and research.

SnackSafely.com snacksafely.com
· Established in 2011, SnackSafely.com provides straightforward, actionable information to help improve the lives of the estimated 32 million people in the United States living with food allergies.

INDEX